The Perfect Practice
for an Efficient Physician

By
Sherry Anderson Delio, MPA, HSA

Published by:
Medical Group Management Association
104 Inverness Terrace East
Englewood CO 80112
(888) 608-5601
Web site: http://www.mgma.com

Medical Group Management Association (MGMA) publications are intended to provide current and accurate information and are designed to assist readers in becoming more familiar with the subject matter covered. Such publications are distributed with the understanding that MGMA does not render any legal, accounting or other professional advice that may be construed as specifically applicable to individual situations. No representation or warranties are made concerning the application of legal or other principles discussed by the authors to any specific factual situation, nor is any prediction made concerning how any particular judge, government official or other person will interpret or apply such principles. Special factual situations should be discussed with professional advisors.

© Copyright 1999
Medical Group Management Association
104 Inverness Terrace East
Englewood CO 80112
ISBN #1-56829-097-7
Item #5336

Table of Contents

Acknowledgments

I would like to dedicate this book to my father – who always encouraged me to do my best.

I would also like to thank my husband Tony, who put up with my many hours at the computer and also my children Monica, Angie and Darin, for all the happiness they bring to our family.

In addition, thanks go to the physicians and staff I work with for all their hard work, and for their patience at trying all the new ideas.

Thanks also to Don Berwick, MD, and all the people at IHI for helping me to look at process improvement in a new light.

My appreciation to Virginia Mason Medical Center, Seattle, and Mercy Family Health Clinic, Phoenix, for sharing their forms.

Special thanks goes to the support of the Medical Group Management Association, especially Cynthia Kiyotake, MS, Director MGMA Library Resource Center. Also sincere appreciation goes to the editorial and production team of: Alys Novak, MGMA Acquisitions Editor; Mary Wayman Huey; Brian Novak; and Network Graphics.

Preface

In 1995, Sherry Delio and George Hein wrote the book *The Making of an Efficient Physician* for the Medical Group Management Association. The book turned out to be MGMA's number one best seller of all times!

Why? The answer is simple. The book lived up to its billing as "down-to-earth, practical and packed with specific ideas and suggestions to build a streamlined, profitable, efficient practice. It is lean, clear, honest, direct and proven." Literally thousands of MGMA members and others in the health care field found this to be true and the book became a classic reference.

The Perfect Practice for an Efficient Physician brings the same gift to medical group administrators, physicians and all others seeking to survive in today's health care environment. Not only does the author update her previous guiding principles for success, but also offers new principles for the new millennium. Once again, the focus is on the essentials that cannot ever be overlooked or underplayed – service standards, operational indicators, simplification, workflow, process, standardization. And once again, the style is right on target: succinct, straightforward, no-nonsense tips that really work!

MGMA is delighted to offer this new classic to its members.

About the author

Sherry Anderson Delio, MPA, HSA, Director of Ambulatory Services of an Arizona medical practice, has been a practice management consultant since 1984 and before that worked as a registered nurse. She holds a master's degree in public administration with an emphasis in health services administration from the University of San Francisco.

Delio, a member of Medical Group Management Association, has measured and analyzed hundreds of physician practices and has researched patient expectations and ambulatory care systems design. She is a frequent presenter to health care groups and is the co-author of the MGMA book, *The Making of an Efficient Physician.*

She has worked on three Institute of Healthcare Initiatives (IHI) related to access and wait time initiatives – one as a participant and two as faculty.

Chapter 1

Introduction

What is happening to health care?

The Making of an Efficient Physician, my previous book, was a down-to-earth guide to running an efficient medical practice. This easy-to-read manual helped physicians understand their daily work life and provided tools and methods for improving their practice. The principles were simple and logical and utilized many of the basic tenets of quality improvement. The approach was "customer driven" and the framework for the "six guiding principles" was based on both observations and time studies of hundreds of physician practices. However, over the past few years, the health care industry has created greater challenges. Reimbursement continues to decrease; costs continue to increase; and managed care continues to regulate health care to a point where it has become one of the most regulated industries in our country. We find ourselves in a system where patients, providers and staff are extremely dissatisfied. Many practices are failing and we must step back and ask ourselves why – what is so different today?

While the six guiding principles stated in the first book, *The Making of an Efficient Physician,* are still the basis for building an efficient and effective practice – what has changed is the medical environment. Having efficient physicians is no longer enough. As workloads increase – expenses must decrease. We must do more with less. The number one question is HOW?

A survival manual for working in today's health care environment

The Perfect Practice for an Efficient Physician looks at today's challenges and identifies opportunities for modifying workflow to develop a sustainable office practice. If we do not help physicians improve their work environment today – they will not be here tomorrow. Life is no longer fun in the office practice. Everyone, including the patients, feels a lack of control. I get calls daily from physicians who really care about their patients but who feel forced to "make the numbers" with less help and more regulations. What they are asking for is a simple manual with easy-to-implement ideas on how to survive in this turbulent environment. Everyone wants to leave at the end of the day feeling accomplished, satisfied and assured that there will be a tomorrow.

Lessons learned from a changing environment

Continued studies of medical practices over the past four years surfaced new issues that were not seen in the past. Increased workload to maintain a positive bottom line continues to create new challenges. Patients' expectations have also changed. They no longer tolerate long waits or poor access. Being seen by their provider of choice on the day they call in has become a standard. Waiting times continue to be the primary complaint of most patients. This results in a need for physicians to increase access while decreasing wait times – a very difficult challenge. Everyone appears dissatisfied with health care today.

This book will update the guiding principles found in *The Making of an Efficient Physician* as well as provide some new guiding principles that will help you in today's environment. Practice size, open access, wait times and workflow in the office are elements that must be addressed to meet the challenges of today. This approach will help improve patient, physician and staff satisfaction, while focusing on the financial viability of the office practice.

Physicians are part of the whole

We used to believe that if we designed systems that allowed our physicians to be as efficient as possible when in the office – the practice would be successful. After all, physicians are the most expensive resource, therefore, if they are efficient – so goes the practice. This is no longer true.

Studies show that the physician's time out of the office is the major barrier to efficient workflow. Efficient workflow allows for increased volumes with decreased resources. Adding additional work to an overly stressed system only results in chaos. Therefore, to add capacity you must first improve the workflow.

Since we have found that physicians are an integral part of all workflow in the office, the physician must spend more time in the office. Adding more staff to compensate for the time physicians are out of the office is no longer feasible. As we talk more about workflow in the book, it will be apparent that physicians drive efficiencies in the office.

Physicians also set the tone for the office staff. The staff will mirror the behavior of the physician. When a physician's tone is negative, the whole structure tends to fall apart. Likewise when physicians are positive and enthusiastic about their work, the staff and patients can sense the tone and are happier with the office environment.

This book will give you suggestions on how physicians can become a central part of the system's workflow. It will give suggestions on measuring flow; identify barriers to flow; and show how adopting some key guiding principles and basic concepts can improve the work environment – thus assuring a sustainable future.

Reimbursement is not improving. In many markets, the outpatient reimbursement continues to tumble. As we see many group practices close their doors, management companies fail and hospitals no longer wanting to financially support physician practices, we must commit to making the changes necessary to develop a viable practice whether standalone or as part of an integrated health care system.

Together we can build a practice that runs smoothly, satisfies patients, retains staff and assures a reasonable level of income for physicians. The challenges are immense and while there often does not seem to be a light at the end of the tunnel, I assure you that following these simple, tried and true principles will be the first step to success. I ask you to take the challenge, spend some time planning your practice using the principles, concepts, tools and methodologies outlined in this book

It will be well worth the 90 minutes or so that it will take to read this book. In particular, recognize that the forms have been time tested with physicians' practices just like yours. Try them, adapt them to your practice – and enjoy the journey.

Chapter 2

What is the "right" size?

What is my panel size?

This is one of the most commonly asked questions in the medical world. You would think from the amount of time spent on determining the ideal panel size that knowing one's panel size must assure success. A panel size is the measurement used today to identify the number of people a particular physician is responsible for. It tends to be the benchmark by which physicians justify their work. It comes from the insurance industry where actuarial tables are used to identify utilization for a population of patients. In 100-percent capitated environments, it is easy to identify the size of each primary care practice, since patients must sign up with a primary care provider, or PCP, who manages their care. By using an age and sex weighted average, it is possible to compare different practices.

Interesting data – but is it information?

In the fee-for-service world or the mixed payer world, it is much more difficult to determine the true size of a practice. The most common methodology for determining a practice, if the practice is less than 55-percent capitated, is to identify the number of unique or different patients seen over an 18-month period. If you run this report every six months, the trend will began to paint a picture of the growth or decline in each practice. By dividing this number into the number of visits, it will show your utilization or the average number of times each patient is seen per 18-month period.

If you have greater than a 55-percent capitated practice, many clinics will extrapolate the utilization rate from the capitated lives and apply that number to the fee-for-service portion of their practice. For example, if you had 1000 capitated lives and from those you saw 2000 visits over a 12-month period, you would have two visits per capitated life. Using the same methodology and knowing that you had 1500 fee-for-service visits, that would equate to 750 equivalent capitated lives. Your panel size would then be 1750 lives.

At the same time it is interesting to run the unique patients by age and sex. Most providers believe they have an older sicker population than others. This usually is not true. Also most practices have an approximate split of 40:60 ratio of men to women in their primary care practice.

Remember it is important that you maintain a well-balanced age distribution in your practice. Often times physicians' practices tend to age as they do and as the years go by, they tend to have a dwindling, older, sicker population which is much more time-consuming and costly to manage.Closing your practice is not an advisable strategy for decreasing your workload.

While these statistics are interesting, are they helpful?

Does knowing your panel size make you successful?

I challenge the notion that identifying the perfect panel size is essential to a successful practice. It is helpful but irrelevant to the success of a practice.

The perfect practice size

A practice is successful when the total costs of resources to give appropriate care, with appropriate outcomes, to a satisfied population is less than or equal to the reimbursement for those services. In other words, a practice is only successful if patients are satisfied and you have a positive bottom line.

How do you determine the appropriate size practice?

Let's look at Dr. Smooth's practice from *The Making of an Efficient Physician*. He wants to know how many visits he needs to see in a year to meet his salary expectations:

- Assume his total expenses are $200,000;

- His desired annual compensation is $150,000;

- Therefore his net revenue requirement would be $350,000;

- If his average net revenue per visit was $100;

- Then the number of encounters (visits) he would need to see to meet his annual compensation requirement would be $350,000/$100 = 3500 visits;

- However, don't forget the no-show rate – assume it is 10 percent;

- Then to net out 3500 visits, he would need to be able to schedule at least 3850 visits.

Next Dr. Smooth wants to know how much time he needs to spend in the office to meet his salary expectations:

- If his average time per visit is 20 minutes;

- His visits per hour are three;

- Then the number of hours he would need to schedule patients would be 3850/3 = 1283 hours per year;

- If the number of weeks he spends in clinic is 45;

- Then Dr. Smooth will need to schedule at least 1283/45 = 28.5 hour per week in the clinic.

However, if his reimbursement were only $50 per visit, he would need twice that amount of time in the office to meet his income expectations. This is where the problem begins.

The number of patients he needs to have in his panel would equate to the number of different patients that would generate the numbers just noted. If he tends to see the same capitated patients more often, his net revenue per visit would decrease, thus resulting in a need to see more different patients. If, on the other hand, he had better utilization and his net revenue per visit increased, he would need a smaller population of patients to meet his compensation expectations.

You can use the same method. Do the math. How many hours do you need to spend in the office?

Total expenses   _____

Desired compensation   _____

Net revenue required   _____

Average minutes/visit   _____

Visit volume required   _____

No-show rate   _____

Scheduled visit volumes   _____

Scheduled hours needed in
clinic to meet volume expectations   _____

Weeks in clinic per year   _____

Average scheduled hours
per week required   _____

This is a somewhat of an oversimplification, however, it is a simple methodology for seeing if it is even possible to meet your expectations. Now that you have a good idea of the length of time you will need to be in the clinic, let's work on making it the most efficient time possible. **Need some help? Read on!!!**

Chapter 3

The guiding principles

Let principles guide your practice

Guiding principles are like road maps that keep everyone moving in the appropriate direction. They take you on the most efficient, effective route to attain your vision. They help in decision-making. No longer are decisions made based on personal needs or expectations. Rather, by using guiding principles, everyone approaches a problem with the same end result in mind. It is a good way to test ideas – do they meet the guiding principles?

Here are the six guiding principles addressed in *The Making of an Efficient Physician:*

- making a time commitment;

- balancing work loads;

- decreasing unnecessary variation;

- distributing tasks appropriately;

- creating a team; and

- allocating resources by volume of work.

This proactive approach focuses on planning ahead – anticipating what may happen. The following is a short overview of each practice management guiding principle.

The first guiding principle is *making a time commitment. Commitment* relates to the amount of time and effort dedicated to seeing patients. It is impossible to build a practice when the physician is not in the office. If there is a mismatch between availability and demand, patient satisfaction will suffer. Too few hours in the clinic normally result in decreased patient volumes and a poor financial future.

The second guiding principle is *balancing workloads.* Smoothing out the peaks and valleys that create high stress will allow physicians to see more patients in less time with greater support and better patient satisfaction. When we talk about demand, we are really talking about the number of patients who want to be seen at a particular time. It used to be true that physicians and staff would determine if it was necessary for the patient to be seen or could be seen on another day. Today, we determine demand by the number of patients requesting an appointment each day. By understanding daily demand, it is possible to shape demand by booking follow-up appointments on low demand days. Example, Mondays tend to be the busiest request day – therefore, on Mondays you would not schedule any follow-up appointments. This will assure that as people call in, they will be seen on that day unless that doesn't meet their needs.

Some HMOs or large practices try to stagger staff and doctors based on the demand. This may work for matching demand and availability – however, it does not help to streamline workflow. Having physicians in clinic five days a week and shaping demand as stated before, will allow a practice to maximize efficiency.

Compliance and consistency improve with standardization. The third guiding principle focuses on *decreasing unnecessary variation.* Variation is costly in many ways. Example: Supply costs increase without a standardized inventory system that identifies a basic set of items that will be used in the clinic. In a group practice it will take the physicians working together to come up with this standard list.

Variation in process results in staff not being able to help each other because they do things so differently.

Variation by providers leaves patients confused. Consistency enhances a patient's confidence in the system.

The fourth principle is *distributing tasks appropriately*. The rule of thumb we use is to delegate to the lowest skill-level person who can safely and legally perform a task. This increases job satisfaction and decreases costs. It also frees up the physician to spend more time with patients. When allowing staff to work at their full potential, it is imperative that you have core competency testing set up annually. It is also imperative that clear policy and procedures are in place, as well as clear job descriptions for each job title. Identifying the scope of practice for each job title is essential. A little knowledge is dangerous. Be sure what your staff do and say what you want them to do and say.

Creating a team – interdependency – is the fifth principle. Many management texts document the advantages of teamwork in the workplace. People working in teams seem to perform more effectively than people working in isolation do. Teamwork enhances communication. Small work units result in the highest functioning teams. Usually teams or pods of four doctors or less work most effectively together. Once the unit is larger than four, communication begins to break down and additional layers of staff are needed to manage the work.

The sixth guiding principle is *allocating resources* by volume of work. A high volume practice needs both more space and support staff than a practice with lower volumes. However, we have found that most high-volume, efficient clinics function best with three staff for every provider. This includes tasks from pre-registration, scheduling, medical records and clinical operations to keying in charges and working the errors. The only tasks not included are transcription, collections and administrative staff.

In the past you would usually find two-thirds of the staff in the front office doing registration, scheduling, check-in, checkout, referrals and billing and only one-third in the back helping the physician. However, we now believe it is far more efficient to have two-thirds of the staff in the back office, closer to the physicians. To move staff to the back, we must also move some of the tasks. We will talk more about re-aligning the office in a later chapter.

Without good customer service – you have nothing

Before we focus on the new guiding principles, we first must review the importance of good customer service. You may have the best systems in the world, however, without good customer service all your hard work will be in vain. It is also not enough that you think you are doing a good job – what is important is that your patients believe you met their needs and perceive the visit to have value. Remember that patients don't care how much you know, until they know how much you care. Don't underestimate the value of good service or the harm poor service can do to your practice.

Chapter 4

Seeing your practice through your patients' eyes

The competitive edge

In the competitive health care environment, customer service is becoming the way in which patients differentiate you from other physicians in your market. Patients, payers and other physicians are evaluating and making health care purchasing decisions based on your ability to meet their needs and expectations. Balancing operational, financial and customer expectations will differentiate you in the marketplace with outstanding service and appropriate care at the right price.

Listen with an empathetic ear

To give good service, you must first learn what the patient and family wants and expects. It is not enough to build a practice based on your own desires – rather ask your patients.

There are four different approaches you can use to identify patients' expectations. The first is to develop a patient satisfaction survey. Keep it simple. No more that ten questions keeps it easy for patients to complete, as well as easy for you to compile the results. A survey will give you general information on how satisfied patients are with the service they received over time. A single survey is not as helpful as periodic samplings of the service. The following is an example of a common patient satisfaction survey used in many clinics today.

Patient Satisfaction Survey

Here are some questions about the visit you just made. In terms of your satisfaction, how would you rate each of the following? Answer each question as honestly as you can. For each question, circle the number associated with the most appropriate response (1, 2, 3, etc.).

Office location_____ Today's Date_____
_____ Physician _____

	Excellent	Very Good	Good	Fair	Poor
1. How long you waited to an appointment	1	2	3	4	5
2. Convenience of the location of the office	1	2	3	4	5
3. Getting through to the office by phone	1	2	3	4	5
4. Length of time waiting at the office	1	2	3	4	5
5. Time spent with the person you saw	1	2	3	4	5
6. Explanation of what was done for you	1	2	3	4	5
7. The technical skills (thoroughness, carefulness, competence) of the person you saw	1	2	3	4	5
8. The personal manner (courtesy, respect, sensitivity, friendliness) of the person you saw	1	2	3	4	5
9. This visit overall	1	2	3	4	5

	Definitely yes	Probably yes	Probably not	Definitely not
10. Would you recommend this physician to your friends and family?				

Comments_____
_____
_____

The second approach is to let your patients help you determine process. This is often times called a *needs assessment.* Before making a change, ask your patients their opinions on the change. One example: If you want to change hours but are not sure what hours your patients would prefer, ask them. You can use a short letter or form. You will be surprised how willing patients are to help you solve your problems.

The third is sometimes more difficult but very effective. Bring together a group of patients to discuss their needs and expectations. These are called *focus groups.* They give you more direct, open-ended input, but are also more time-consuming. However, there is no substitute for actively listening to patients. It is amazing how easy it is to satisfy patients if you are respectful of their needs and show them that you truly care about their well-being.

The fourth is to ask your patients to *write a letter* about their ideal office visit. This is a great technique to really involve your patients in your practice. The following is a sample.

My ideal patient visit

My ideal visit would start when I called to arrange for care. The phone rang twice and was answered by a very pleasant person who seemed eager to help me. She was courteous and asked how she could help. I related that I was a new patient and she offered an appointment with the physician at 2 p.m. today. She also stated that she was arranging for me to meet with the manager 15 minutes before my appointment to establish me with the practice. She reminded me of the information I needed to bring in, including all of my medications and insurance card. She even thanked me for choosing this health center.

I arrived at 1:35 p.m. and was greeted by a very friendly person who seemed genuinely pleased to see me. She escorted me back to the manager's office. I didn't have to sit and wait in the lobby. The manager asked for my insur-

ance card and put all the information into the computer. She explained how they collect co-pays at the front desk and how the billing system works. It was very nice to do this in the privacy of her office. She also explained how to access the practice after hours and gave me a list of numbers to call if I needed anything in the future. She welcomed me into the practice and walked me out and introduced me to the physician's staff.

The medical assistant asked me for my medications, collected the appropriate information, gave me a gown and stated that the doctor would be right in.

As soon as I was ready, the physician walked in. He was very friendly, asked me if I had any problems and then proceeded to listen until I was finished talking. He seemed really interested. He answered all my questions, did the physical exam and then talked to me about his findings and his suggestions. As we were talking, he wrote down what he was ordering. He also asked me how I would like my results returned and I stated, if the results were normal, a letter would be fine. If not, I would appreciate a phone call to my home. He asked me to get dressed and informed me that the medical assistant would be in to draw my blood.

As soon as I was dressed, the assistant came in and drew my blood, handed me some educational information and walked me out and introduced me to the desk assistant and handed her the paperwork.

The desk assistant was very helpful. She went over my orders to make sure I understood everything the doctor told me. I needed a referral to the dermatologist so she called, got the referral and then called and made an appointment for me. She also made my follow-up appointment and keyed in my charges so I was aware before I left of exactly what I owed. She then gave me a copy of the order sheet to help me remember what the doctor ordered along with the time of my next appointment and the appointment with the dermatologist. She thanked me for coming in and let me know I would be getting a letter within a week if all my tests were normal – if not, I would get a call from the doctor immediately.

I left feeling very special. The letter arrived a week after my visit just as they promised. I was fine – and felt fine about my experience.

Much can be learned about what is important to this patient through her letter. It pays to encourage patients to write. Given them a prepaid return envelope to make it easy, as well as simple instructions on the type of information you seek.

Be courteous and helpful

It is amazing how a smile, eye contact, and kind words can make the difference between a positive and a negative experience for the patient, regardless of the clinical findings.

Always address patients by name. Introduce yourself and be sure that everyone wears a name tag with at least their first name and title large enough so elderly patients can read it. Ask patients if they would prefer a family member to join in the discussion. Let it be the patient's decision.

Help the patient be prepared

It is very uncomfortable for patients to come in without the needed information. They are frequently angry at the clinic for not informing them of what they needed to bring in when they made their appointment. If they don't know their insurance company, what medications they are on, or don't have a list of their child's immunizations, it may start the visit off negatively.

Never make patients wait

This has become the number one patient complaint in the past few years. Patients are now shopping for doctors who have easy access and little or no wait. Remember that situations may arise that throw you off schedule, so have a contingency plan. Be respectful of their time and they will be respectful of yours.

Give the patients time to tell their story

It only takes about two minutes for a patient to tell his/her story. Listen carefully and you will find that the visit is much shorter than it would be if you didn't "invite" the story right upfront. When they seem to be finished, be sure they are. Patients usually start with the least significant issue and work toward the most serious concerns. When physicians interrupt to address each issue separately, they usually run out of time and when you are ready to leave the room, the patient brings up the real reason for the visit. This causes delays and makes patients feel like they are being rushed. Try being quiet for two minutes. It is not easy – but it works!

Put it in writing

Patients remember about 30 percent of what you tell them during their visit. If you will write down your treatment plan, patients will leave more satisfied, compliance will improve and you will have fewer calls back to the office to verify the plan. Patients also like walking out with something in hand.

Timely follow-up

No news is good news is no longer acceptable. Patients want to know the results of all tests as soon as possible. Having test verification and results reporting procedures is imperative. We will discuss this in a later chapter.

A courtesy phone call to check on a patient's condition will win you a patient for life. These proactive calls take very little time, yet make a patient feel very special.

Most patients have similar expectations. What helps a patient feel value is also what helps us be efficient. While easy access, short waits, knowledge and expertise at fair price are expectations today, courtesy and respect with a helpful attitude will leave patients espousing your greatness to all who will listen.

A word about how attitude affects lawsuits

It is not always just a bad outcome that sends a patient to an attorney. What physicians and/or staff members say or do can prevent or trigger a claim or a suit. Many people change doctors because they are dissatisfied with the attitude of the office, not the care. The quality of interaction between patient and staff appears to underlie the patient's evaluation of the overall quality of care. Most malpractice claims stem from patients' feelings about how they were treated – not the actual care that was given.

The easiest way to meet all of these expectations is to do the appropriate things the appropriate way the first time!

Chapter 5

Service standards and operational indicators

Building the framework

Service standards, operational indicators and patient satisfaction surveys are all tools that will help you manage your practice. Share this information with your staff. Use the information to help identify weaknesses in your practice, but also use the information when it is positive to reward your staff. Make sure staff are working with you to improve your practice.

Service standards

Service standards are one way of describing appropriate service. They set the framework for your staff. We all have different ideas as to what good service means. So be clear, write down your service standards so your staff will be clear as to how you expect your patients to be treated.

There are nine elements to consider when determining if you are doing the right thing:

- Efficacy – Did the action achieve the desired outcome?

- Appropriateness – Is the action appropriate under the circumstances?

- Availability – Is it available to the patient?

- Timeliness – Is it done in a timely manner, which meets the patient's expectation?

- Effectiveness – Is it completed in a beneficial manner?

- Continuity – Is there consideration as to how the next steps will be performed?

- Safety – Is it a safe environment for the patient?

- Efficiency – Is there a relationship between the care and the resources needed?

- Respect and caring – Is the patient involved and is confidentiality assured?

The following are a few examples of how to put these standards to work to please the patient.

Telephone service standards

- Answer all calls within three rings.

- Return all calls within one hour.

- Document all calls in the medical record.

- Always identify yourself and ask, "How may I help you?"

- Be cheerful.

- Speak clearly, but in a low tone of voice to avoid being overheard.

Remember telephone effectiveness is 82 percent voice tone and quality and only 18 percent the words we say. Teach your staff how to talk on the phone, not just what words to say. Make sure patients can feel the smile on your staff's face.

Verbal communication standards

- Be positive and friendly.

- Greet with a "Hello. How are you?" Express a personal interest.

- Establish eye contact when speaking and acknowledge the patient.

- Smile.

- Wear your name badge.

- Maintain a neat, clean and professional appearance.

- Your working area and all public working areas should be kept neat, clean and professional.

- Keep people informed – if an appointment is running late – tell them, update often so they do not feel forgotten.

Communication effectiveness is only 7 percent the words we say; 38 percent how we say it; and 55 percent visual, body language. Body language counts. Several clinics I have worked with have videotaped the staff so they can actually see how their behavior affects the patient's behavior. It is a great learning tool.

Operational indicators help measure your success

It is also important for your staff to understand by which operational indicators you are measuring the clinic's performance. There are several categories of indicators. It is important to measure your performance against benchmarks, but also to measure your performance to monitor improvement. A good source for benchmark data would be MGMA. The following list is a sample of some of the more important indicators.

Productivity indicators

- Annual visits (office, hospital, other);

- Annual RVUs;

- Hours in clinic; and

- Square foot per physician.

Staff and operating performance indicators

- Cycle time (length of time from check-in through checkout);

- Wait times – there are several wait states in a cycle: wait for the phone to be answered, wait to get an appointment, wait in the lobby, wait in the exam room, wait for referral, wait for results, etc. They are all important to focus on. It is important to monitor cycle time as you work on wait times, because improving one wait time may produce an increase in the wait time in another area of your system;

- No-show and same-day cancel rates;

- Delays in payment posting;

- Denial rates; and

- Days in account receivable.

Patient satisfaction indicators

- Overall satisfaction;

- Percent who recommend physician or group; and

- Disenrollment rate.

Physician performance indicators

- Coding accuracy;

- Charge recovery;

- Chart audits;

- Patient call backs; and

- On-call patient response.

Poor performance is costly

Remember, of the people who are dissatisfied, only 4 percent will complain; 96 percent go away; and of those, 91 percent never come back. Also one unhappy person will tell at least eight others. However, 70 percent of the people will come back if the complaint is resolved and 95 percent will come back if the complaint is resolved on the spot. Poor service is time-consuming and costly. We spend far more time on trying to attract new business than to keep the old. Spend more time satisfying your existing patients. Measuring performance is a key to understanding where you should spend your time improving your practice.

How will you know you have achieved outstanding service?

You will no longer have to take time to apologize for patient waits or poor service. The "waiting room" will be a thing of the past and waits, delays and extra steps will be eliminated. This will allow you more time to take care of the patients' medical needs.

The original guiding principles focused on helping the physician become as efficient as possible. The new guiding principles in the following chapter will help to set the tone by which your office will operate.

Chapter 6

New guiding principles

Guiding principles that affect the culture of your organization

The following eight guiding principles relate to the cultural norms of your organization. These help your staff better understand the spirit by which you expect your office to function.

Build an efficient practice around the needs of the patient

The first guiding principle relates to customer service. Understanding your patients' needs is even more critical than in years past. You must set the tone in your office to be patient focused. Before implementing any change, you must ask, "How will this affect my patients"? If it does not add value, reconsider the change. Two of the greatest gifts you can bring to your practice are your sincerity and your genuine interest in your patients as people.

Simplification

Simplification is the second guiding principle. Go back to basics. Health care has become far too complicated. We take a fairly easy process and turn it into a chaotic nightmare for many patients. After all, what a patient desires is to call, get an appointment, come in and see the physician, walk out with a treatment plan and be given the results of the tests in a realistic timeframe. Sounds pretty straight-forward – but for most patients it is far from an easy process.

Be proactive

Being reactive or passive no longer works in this health care environment. The third guiding principle addresses the need to be proactive. Give your staff the latitude to right any wrongs. In other words, if a patient has a complaint, let the staff resolve the problem on the spot. Make it an expectation that if a patient has a concern, whoever is helping that person will resolve the issue. None of this, "It's not my job," or passing patients around like a football. Be proactive – fix it!

Real-time work – do today's work today

If there is one thing you take away from reading this book, it should be the fourth guiding principle. Real-time work is by far the key to efficiency. Batching your work to do at a later time is the cause of most delays and frustration in any work environment.

I like to use the analogy of washing dishes. While preparing dinner, if you rinse off the bowls, pots and pans and put them in the dishwasher as you complete the preparation, the only tasks you have left to do is clear the table. When dinner is completed, it only takes a few minutes to rinse off the dishes, put them in the dishwasher, wipe down the table and maybe sweep the floor. You are done. It took you only five to ten minutes to complete the task.

However, if you stack the bowls, pots, pans and dishes in the sink to do the next morning, it will take you at least 30 minutes or more.

This increased your task time by 20 minutes. It also caused you to take time away from today to do a task when you had the time to do the task yesterday. This is what frustrates your staff. Coming to work knowing that most of your day is already filled with work from the previous day is worrisome at best. "How will I ever be able to handle the work that comes in today?" is a question I often hear from staff. It is overwhelming!

This is also true for physicians. When your schedule is full before you even start your day, you must wonder how you will ever see the patients who need to be seen today. Normally patients get backed up in your schedule further and further. We will discuss a solution – Open Access – in another chapter.

There are very few tasks that cannot be completed on the same day. Too often we separate out steps of a task and turn them into a separate task. One example is filing. Many clinics hire medical records staff to do nothing but file loose papers. With the number of people who touch that piece of paper, it is amazing that no one can file it in the chart. It is not uncommon to see staff send both the loose filing and the chart back to medical records so the medical records staff can do the filing. This is what we consider non-value-added work. It is costly and time-consuming.

Referrals are an example of creating a separate job in the process that slows down the workflow. Doing referrals should be part of the discharge assistance tasks. When it is moved off line and done by a separate person, delays are created and service diminishes.

Charge entry is an example of a task that is often times batched, yet should be done at the time of the visit. It is commonly completed at a later time and often in another area. In many clinics it has become a separate function. This results in an increased error rate and/or billing cycle delays.

Batching work not only creates delays, it also increases costs by requiring additional staff and space.

Do it right the first time – avoid rework

Do it right the first time is the fifth guiding principle. The saying, "If you don't have time to do it right, how will you find time to do it over?" is so true. Slow down and complete each task correctly. It really takes no longer to do it right than it does to do it wrong. In health care we actually have developed a department that does nothing but rework – rebillers. That certainly speaks to the inherent inefficiencies in health care today. I am always amazed at the number of times we touch the same piece of paper; answer a call from the same patient; or fax the same form to an insurance company because someone in the process did not complete the task correctly the first time.

Lean thinking

Lean thinking is the sixth guiding principle. Basically lean thinking provides us with a way to think about how we can do more and more with less and less. It helps us look at processes that consume less human effort, less equipment, less time and less space while focusing on meeting the needs of the patients. It is not about destroying jobs in the name of efficiency. It is about looking at every task and asking, "Does it add value?" Then take every step in that task and ask the same question. You are looking to wipe out waste; eliminate tasks or steps of tasks that do not add value.

Look at your practice as a system. Within this system you see patients, which we call encounters. Within each encounter there are several functions. In this book we will refer to three main functions: intake, process and output. Each of these functions has multiple tasks of which there are multiple steps. One example could be weighing the patient, which is a step in the rooming task. This task is part of the process function.

When referring to lean thinking, we are looking at how we can better understand the system. Flow diagramming each function is an easy tool to use. Look for value in each step. Also look for waste. Remove the steps that do not add value.

Continuous flow

Once you have identified all the value-added steps necessary to complete the encounter, you must determine the most efficient flow. The seventh guiding principle addresses the need for continuous flow rather than batching work to do later. It was once thought that performing like tasks in batches was most efficient. An example is when physicians batch their charts to dictate at the end of the day. Time studies have shown that it takes three to five times longer to dictate if done at the end of the day than if done in a continuous flow during or after seeing each patient.

While we know batching work results in long delays, it also discourages multitasking. Multitasking has been found to decrease resource costs. The solution is continuous flow. Complete all steps of each task before moving on to the next.

Working in small work units

The eighth guiding principle is working in small work units. Large centralized systems have inherent communication problems. The people performing the tasks are so far removed from the patient that they lose perspective of the patient's needs. Everyone begins to work in silos, losing sight of the mission of the organization. Look at the mission statements of the different departments. How many of them even mention patients? Centralized functions also create the need for increased supervision, which adds cost to the system.

Moving the work closer to the patient/physician interaction has proven to decrease costs as well as increase patient, physician and staff satisfaction. It allows for decreased rework, increased communication and decreased costs. We will discuss a staffing model that moves the work closer to the patient/physician interaction in a later chapter,

Make it a way of life

Patient focused, lean thinking, continuous flow and small work units are all intertwined and need to be the way of life in your office. Making sure you and your staff take the time to do the right things the right way the first time, and to complete all of today's tasks today will all help in moving you toward a more positive future. You must walk the talk.

System thinking

Think of your practice as a system. For the purpose of this book, when we talked about "lean thinking," we discussed the system as the encounter. Within the system we have three functions: intake, process and output. Intake is actually the preparation function. Several tasks are covered in the preparation phase, including but not limited to scheduling, registration, visit preparation and check-in. The second function is process. Included in this function are activities related to the reason for the visit. Some of the tasks included in this phase are rooming, time with the physician, immunizations, procedures, etc. Output becomes the follow-up phase. Included in this phase are such tasks such as check-out, test verification, results reporting, charge entry, referrals and follow-up. We will address each function in more detail in another chapter.

Chapter 7

Space versus workflow

Form follows function

A word about designing your office. Poorly designed space can be very costly. The size of the space is not as important as the functionality. Take the time to analyze both paper and patient flow to assure that you designed an efficient and effective floor plan. Here are some basic concepts to consider when designing medical office space:

- Small work units;

- Maximum flexibility;

- Small waiting room to discourage long waits;

- Optimal communication;

- Circular flow;

- Optimal visibility;

- Confidentiality; and

- Minimal distance between tasks.

Generic rooms allow any physician the ability to work out of any room at any time. This adds great flexibility. Staff are able to use rooms interchangeably, which will increase throughput and guarantee that rooms never become the constraint.

Small work units

Even in a large clinic, the concept of small work units makes sense. The ability to move staff and functions closer to the patient/physician interaction allows the physician to take a more active role in the entire encounter.

The following floor plan adopts many of the concepts just listed. This clinic was built out for three physicians and a nurse case manager. The physician and staff in this clinic find it very functional and a patient-friendly floor plan that enhances communication and multitasking. It also encourages real-time work, since no space was built out for batch work to do at a later time.

Floor Plan

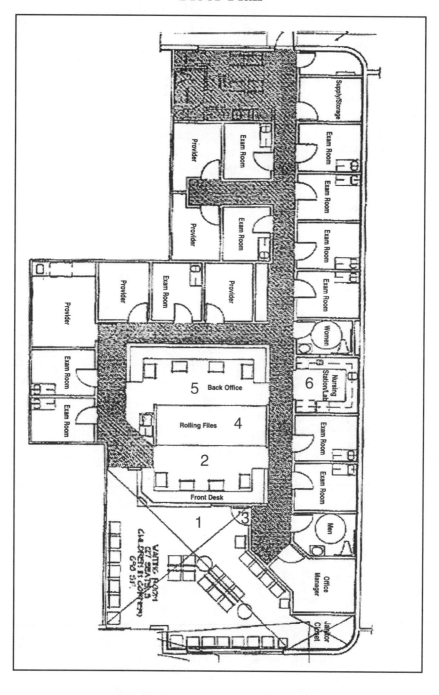

If we were to rebuild this floor plan again, we would decrease the waiting room (1). It appeared smaller on the plans, however, once it was built and since we have very short wait times, we would prefer to add the space to the back office.

The front desk (2) is open, without a glass window to separate the patients from the staff. We have learned from talking to patients that glass partitions separating them from the staff are dissatisfiers. We wanted an open, friendly place to greet our patients.

Patients enter to the right of the front desk (3). They are weighed next to the door which is away from the other staff and patients. The exam rooms and physicians' offices surround the workstation.

The key to improving the communication was to have a single work area for both the front and back office staff, separated by rolling medical records (4). The medical records between the front and the back act as a barrier so patients cannot see or hear what is going on in the back office (5). However, because of the aisles between the files, staff are able to easily communicate. With medical records in the center, all staff are responsible for the medical record tasks. By giving the staff headphones, they are able to retrieve or refile medical records while doing other tasks.

Each physician has three exam rooms with his/her office close by. The nursing station (6) where immunizations, supplies, etc., are stored is across the hall from the major work area. Staff are trained on how to maintain confidentiality in an open work area. Because of being able to adopt the continuous flow principle, patients are not left waiting in any area.

Minimizing hand-offs was another concept we adopted. Many systems require that patients be transferred to multiple people, offices or workstations to complete the processing or service. The hand-off from one stage to the next can cause increased time and costs and cause quality problems. We tried to rearrange the workflow to minimize hand-off during the encounter. Each job was expanded to take on multiple tasks. Another concept we used was to make sure everyone was cross-trained to as many tasks as possible. Everyone must handle multiple tasks rather than be specialist in one specific area.

What makes a team work well

Clarity of purpose and knowing that they will be active participants in process improvement will help staff feel part of the team. By being fair to all, honest in everything you do and consistent, your staff will build trust in you and the organization. Communication is the key to a productive staff. It is amazing how much more productive happy people are than employees who hate their job.

Staffing model

We re-aligned our staffing model to reflect the three functions of our system. We have one office assistant in the front doing the intake function for each full-time physician. We now have two medical assistants in the back doing the process and output functions for each full-time physician. The only registered nurses in any of the clinics are case managers, who function as providers of care.

This allows both paper flow and patient flow to continue at the same time. The process medical assistant is the person who rooms the patient and assists the physician with any procedures. The output medical assistant is responsible for all the paperwork and follow-up. Many of the tasks of this person are tasks that were previously done in the front office. By moving them to the back, we were able to better support the physicians without adding staff.

Involve staff in understanding workflow

Pull your team together and clarify the mission so everyone is in agreement on your purpose. Identify the key functions and develop high-level flowcharts for each.

Identify areas of concern in each function and begin a process improvement project.

Practice assessment

Ask each staff member to follow a patient through your system. Help your staff better understand what a patient goes through trying to access care. Staff in the back office don't have a good understanding of some of the barriers in the front office. The opposite is also true. It is also important that the physicians walk through the system with a patient. Much can be learned about the barriers to care by observing the total system. Use the following Practice Assessment Tool during these walk-throughs.

Practice Assessment Tool

1. Do the clinic hours meet the patients' needs?

2. Do you open up your phone lines at least a half-hour before the clinic opens?

3. How long does the patient wait in the lobby?

4. Is the check-in process confidential?

5. Do staff collect co-pays and any balance due at time of check-in?

6. How many stops does a patient need to make during the encounter?

7. How long does the patient wait in the exam room before the physician comes in?

8. Did the patient bring in his/her insurance card?

9. Did the patient bring in all current medications?

10. Was the room ready for the patient?

11. Did the physician have to leave the room to retrieve any items?

12. Are all rooms interchangeable?

13. Was all the loose filing up to date?

14. Are there clear rooming criteria for specific patient appointments?

15. Are follow-up appointments made in the back office?

16. Was the referral done or at least started while the patient was in the office?

17. Were the charges keyed in before the patient left the office?

18. Does a different person collect the money than the one who keys in the charges?

19. Does the deposit have two signatures?

This is a sample of the types of questions you want to have available when you or your staff observe your system for a day. Be sure to ask questions that relate to doing the appropriate task at the appropriate time the correct way.

You will be amazed at the number of problems that surface each day. Insufficient capacity or inability to do real-time work will most likely be the cause of most of the problems that surface during your observation. The next chapter will address the insufficient capacity issue.

Chapter 8

Open access

Patients' access expectation

To be seen when they want to be seen, by the provider of choice!

Access problems

Poor access to care is a major concern in health care today. It is not uncommon for a patient to call for an appointment and not be seen for weeks, which results in unnecessary visits to emergency rooms or urgent care clinics. Many of the workflow problems we experience every day are a result of poor access.

Inability to get through on the phones is often times caused by poor access. Talk time on the phone increases as access decreases, since it takes longer to schedule an appointment when you have limited availability. Sometimes it even generates a call to the back office or a message that needs to be returned to the patient at another time – all non-value-added rework.

The cost is great! Don't measure the loss in dollars alone but in the damage it does to your reputation. Many patients leave practices because of poor access, even if they are happy with the care of the physician.

No-show rates increase the further out you schedule patients. To compensate, clinics end up adding the task of calling to remind patients of their visit – again another non-value-added task which adds unnecessary costs to the system.

An open access system assures that all patients will be seen on the day they call. Of course, if the patient requests a different day, then he/she is scheduled the day requested.

One of the basic tenets of an open access system is that physicians will see their own patients. Two major physician satisfiers of this system are the fact that physicians get to see their own patients and those patients no longer complain about poor access.

There are many ways to move to an open access system. The first step is to make the commitment. It is hard work and at times very worrisome. Those days when you come to work and the schedule is extremely light are frightening. However, every practice that I have seen that has gone to an open access system has increased their productivity.

If you have a backlog, you must make the commitment to gain capacity. One way to create future capacity is to do all today's work today. It may mean that you will need to have some very long days for a week or two. However, the backlog will end and you will be glad you made the sacrifice because life in an open access system is so much better.

Some people will choose a date and just begin open access as of that day by staying as late as it takes to see all the patients who want to be seen each day. This works well if you do not have a large backlog of patients. However, if you are determined to improve your work life, even with a large backlog, I highly recommend this method.

Many doctors, however, choose to carve out more and more time each week until they have between 30-50 percent of their schedule open to same-day visits. It works, but until you are willing to have that flexible end of day, you will never reap the full benefit of an open access system.

Appointment types

Once you decide to move to an open access system, it is imperative that you simplify your appointment types. We chose to have one appointment length based on the average time of all visits. After collecting data for over a year, we were able to determine that an average time of 20 minutes per visit would allow for the number of visits needed per year as well as an even workflow through the clinic. The even workflow is equally as important as the time a physician needs to see the patient. Granted there are many patients who could be seen in less time. However, to bring patients in at a faster pace than every 20 minutes, added undue stress to the rest of the system. Remember we were also expecting the staff to complete each task real time.

After deciding to adopt the philosophy of a singular appointment time based on the average length of time per visit, we had to identify the reasons for some visits taking more than the average time. During our study we noted that the two major reasons for patients taking longer than average were poor historical information available or the patients were poor communicators and usually had multiple problems. By using the technique of letting the patients talk until they completed telling their story before interrupting and assuring that all paperwork was in the chart and ready, most patients were seen within the time allotted. By planning ahead, having translators in place if necessary and having everything ready for the physician, we were able to go to one appointment time for all patients in primary care. Specialty care still prefers two times. The shorter visits gave the physicians the opportunity to catch patients up on their health maintenance, if appropriate, or to complete paperwork or call-backs.

During our study to transition to an open access system, we chose to use four appointment types, all 20 minutes in length. Our objective was to see if bringing patients in at even intervals would improve process time. It allowed everyone to work at a more even pace and amazingly, we were able to increase the throughput of patients.

To better understand your patient demand, try using the following four appointment types. Use *dr. request* for all appointments requested by the physician after a visit. The number of these appointments is important because it will help you identify the percent of your practice that will be filled in advance. *Patient request* is used when an appointment was requested, same day was available, but the patient preferred another day. These are the only two visit types that should be prescheduled. The remainder of the patients should be seen on the *same day,* which is the third appointment type. The fourth type is *no match,* which means we did not meet the patient's needs. This is an important indicator to measure over time. While the appointment types do not specify what the patient is coming in for, the comments do. Each appointment needs a reason for the visit annotated to help the staff prepare for the visit.

This works well when you are in clinic, however, there will be times when you are out of clinic for various reasons. Make a contingency plan. When you are out of the office or need to leave early one day, how will you compensate for the demand that is moved to a future day? Also if your practice is financially doing well and you have more patients than you can possibly care for – what is your plan? Nice problem to have!!

You may want to look at decreasing patient demand. Some ways of reducing demand are to handle patient issues over the phone. Some physicians are actually using e-mail to communicate with their patients. Group visits are working in some areas. OB and geriatrics seem to be two areas conducive to group visits. Are you seeing your patients back more often than necessary? Are you taking advantage of each visit to do all that you can to reduce the need for another visit? These are some ideas on how you can reduce your demand.

Smoothing demand is important especially in areas where demand fluctuates widely at different times of the year, month, week or day. Rather than trying to flex staff to handle the peak demands, steps can often be taken to better distribute the demand. If summers are slow, encourage your healthy patients to come in for their routine exams in the summer. Patients will appreciate knowing that they will be better served in the summer when all the acute illness patients are not in the clinic. Likewise, if there is a day of the week that is busier with requests, decrease the number of pre-appointed visits on that day. Work with your schedule. Understand your demand and manage your availability.

Chapter 9

Waits and delays

Constraints

I would define a constraint as an inability to get work done effectively and efficiently in a smoother manner – the first time and without delays. Constraints are often times referred to as bottlenecks within a system. They are the rate-limiting step in all systems. Every system has at least one predominant constraint. While it is important that you identify the constraints, it is more important that you learn how to manage them. A system is like a chain. As long as the integrity is maintained, the chain works well. However, as soon as one link in the chain is defective or weak, so goes the functionality of the chain. It is no different in your office. As long as every task within the system is done appropriately, the system works well. However, there are hundreds of circumstances that appear daily to interrupt the flow.

If there is a single constraint in your system, it should be the physician. Therefore, you must focus on optimizing the physician's time. Usually the physician's schedule becomes a major constraint in most systems. When this happens, throughput is limited because the physician's schedule is full and patients are put off until another day. This constraint is costly.

People do not always cause constraints. Space, equipment, or even outdated or erroneous policies can be the source

Focus on maximizing throughput while minimizing operational expense. As you walk through your system, look for areas that limit the flow. Identify why the flow is slowed or stopped at a particular place. What could be done to eliminate the delay? Does eliminating the delay cause another delay further down the process?

In the office practice, waits become major constraints. Throwing more resources at the constraint will not necessarily resolve the problem. Too many different people involved in any system results in increased chaos. Communication breaks down. We have also noted that when we add too many resources to a process, no more work is accomplished. Too much time is wasted on hand-offs and unnecessary communication. No one seems to know who is doing what. Again we must look at simplification.

Referrals are a good example of adding additional staff to do only referrals. They never seemed to get completed in a timely manner and were generating a tremendous amount of extra work. Patients were calling in requesting updates on the status of their referral. Of course the only person who knew the answer was the referral person and if she was out, the whole process stopped. When we transition this task back to the back office, all the rework was eliminated and the referrals were done on the day of the visit. We reduced the waste by reducing the number of people interacting with the process and the patient.

One way of decreasing costs is to maximize throughput. Cutting staff for the sake of cutting cost without identifying the constraints in your system is counterproductive.

Don't forget to look at the systems that support your encounter, like your inventory system. Supplies can become the constraint in your system.

Inventory system

Key concepts, which allow you to maintain a "just in time" inventory system, include appropriate inventory on hand and decreased cost of goods. Inventory is expensive; however, there is also a cost when supplies are a constraint. As you develop your relationship with vendors, look for a vendor that will help you optimize capital, reduce expenditures, provide for standardization and increase service levels. A good vendor should allow you to shorten the supply chain by eliminating redundant costs and duplicate activities, including multiple invoicing and vendor payment tasks.

Negotiate with your vendor a program that will implement cost controls, which will reduce your costs of equipment and supply expenditures immediately. A greater percentage of reduction will be accomplished by ongoing partnerships with your vendors. Many vendors have web-based software which will return the purchasing management control to you. They allow you to: create and send orders; maintain an order on file; view pricing and contracts; receive confirmations; and maintain inventory/par levels. They also allow you to print easy-to-understand reports.

By maintaining appropriate par levels and ordering weekly, you will be assured of not overstocking or running out of needed supplies. Too often support staff identify items that need to be ordered when you run out. This last-minute ordering may be more costly. On the other hand, I often see large quantity of supplies taking up valuable space.

Many times old supplies are discarded. Controlling inventory costs is an easy way to reduce operational expense.

Reducing delays and wait times

Redesign your system to reduce delays. There are several concepts, some of which we have already discussed, that you can use to help decrease wait times in your office.

Do tasks in parallel. By having one medical assistant help to move the patient through the system and the other moving paperwork, neither is being delayed. Physicians can be seeing one patient while the medical assistant prepares the next.

Start on time. There is nothing more frustrating than starting your day off late. If you consistently start late, reconsider your starting time. It is not fair to your patients or staff to continually start late.

Move steps closer together. By adopting the staffing model we talked about, you will gain greater support from your team.

Use automation. Take advantage of any opportunity to automate your system. I have several physicians trying out a voice-activated documentation system. The technology is there; the ease of using it needs a little work. However, this technology will certainly help to decrease costs of transcription. Another automated system that has worked well is the results reporting system.

Minimize the hand-offs. Limit the number of different people your patients need to interact with during their visit. The more interactions, the more complicated the visit becomes.

Synchronize patient, physician and information. Agree that everything will be in the room and ready at the time of the visit. In every clinic I have studied, over 75 percent of the patients come early to their appointments. Don't wait to start the process until the time of the visit. If the patient is there, start the process.

Eliminate anything that is not used. Clean out drawers, cupboards, rooms, etc. Excess clutter slows down your system. Make sure you have a place for everything that is needed and everything is always in the appropriate place. Label all the shelves for easy inventory control. You would be amazed at how much time is wasted looking for supplies or equipment.

Promote self-care by encouraging your patients to purchase one of the books on what to do at home before calling your doctor. There are several good books used by many physicians. It is even helpful to have several in your office to show your patients how to use. A little time spent teaching the patient how to use the book may save many future phone calls.

Walk the talk

The next three chapters will walk you through the functions of an office visit. Remember the guiding principles as we review the tasks within each function of our office practice system.

Chapter 10

Intake

Front office tasks

The intake function incorporates all of the access tasks. Included in this function are such tasks as scheduling, check-in, registration, eligibility and authorizations, medical records preparation, and message calls. The intent is to do all tasks that are at the front end of the system. Tasks from the back end of the system are never done in the front office, because they will cause a delay in the intake function.

Technology – a blessing and a curse

We are in the technology age where what we need to make life easier is out there, but most of us cannot afford to implement a total integrated system. So we are left with bits and pieces that sometimes help and often times complicate our lives. Keep the advantages and disadvantages in mind as you consider these technological tools.

Telephone systems

Telephone systems are extremely sophisticated today. However, most people are only aware of their basic functionality and do not use their systems to the fullest potential. Your telephone system is normally not what causes phone problems, but rather the way the phone system is used. Too often the utilization of our phone systems inhibits patient access to care. Let the representative from your phone system help you better understand how the functionality of the phone can help you meet your patients' needs.

Key concepts to remember:

- Develop service standards as we talked about earlier in this book.

- To staff phones appropriately, data on volumes, handling times, hold times, wait times, abandoned calls and service levels are necessary.

- ACD – automated call distribution system – is a feature of a single phone number/line which, when called, puts callers into a queue. From the queue (or holding area), each call is sent to the next available staff member according to the order in which the call was received. This may help to improve telephone service but must be staffed appropriately or patients will have long waits.

- Access to appointments is inversely related to the amount of time spent handling a call. When access is poor, handling time increases. If handling time increases, hold/wait times increase.

- Identify the top five reasons for phone calls. Your goal should be to decrease non-value-added or unnecessary telephone calls.

- Everyone should be able to answer phones and make appointments. The flow of calls is variable, therefore, the number of staff on the phone must vary with demand.

- Headphones allow your staff to handle larger numbers of calls in a shorter period of time without work injuries.

Telephone communication

One of the most common ways to communicate with patients is by telephone. However, you must carefully assess the level of professionalism of the staff members who have direct contact with patients and/or other health care providers. The greater the level of independence of the staff member interacting with the patient, the greater the liability exposure is. Of even greater significance is the independence granted to the staff member in triaging telephone calls. The physician, driven by patients' needs and defined by appropriate policies and protocols, must direct the level of triage.

All telephone communication should be directly entered or transcribed into the patient's record. It should be treated as part of the patients' clinical information and retained under the same rules as the medical record.

Message taking

- The following information should be documented on all messages:

- Date and time of call;

- Patient's name and age;

- Nature of patient's concern/complaint;

- History;

- Intervention;

- Follow-up; and

- Signature of individual documenting the message (the following two samples have been used very effectively in medical practices).

Messages

Date_____   ___Urgent

Chart #_____   ___Routine

TO:_____Time msg. taken:_____Time msg. delivered_____

Patient name:_____DOB:_____Insurance_____

Provider:_____PCP:_____

Call back #:_____Pharmacy #:_____Allergies:_____

URGENT

___Sudden abdominal pain   ___Sudden back pain

___Sudden eye pain   ___Sudden joint pain/swelling

___Nausea   ___Diarrhea (blood, mucous)

___Recent injury swelling   ___Bloody urine

___Decreased amount of urine   ___Difficulty urinating

___Vomiting and diarrhea (24 hours+)   ___Temp_____(always ask)

___Decreased appetite and/or fluids (older than 75)

ROUTINE

___Cough, congestion, earache   ___Burning with urination

___Headache, sinus drainage   ___Constipation (24 hours+)

___Lab and x-ray results   ___Pain management

___Prescription refills   ___Referral request

___Hives, rash, swelling (no difficulty breathing)

___Temp_____(always ask)

Message taken by:_____

Action Taken By Nurse

___Notified provider   ___Same day appointment   ___Prescription to pharmacy

___Allergies

Comments:_____

_____

_____

_____

Nurse initials_____Provider signature_____Date:_____

Patient Encounter Form

Social Security number:_____

Date:_____Time:_____
Phone(H):_____(W)_____

Problem:_____
_____
_____
_____
_____

Allergies:_____
Meds:_____
Pregnant: _____yes _____no
Pharmacy phone #:_____
Name:_____

CL#_____MD_____

Assessment/Advice:_____
_____
_____
_____
_____

Follow up:_____
_____
_____
_____
_____

Medical record
Insert in chart_____ CSF_____

_____
(signature)

From Virginia Mason Medical Center, Seattle. Used with permission.

Don't forget to document in the chart all after-hours calls. Also when using the telephone to communicate test results, you must document:

• Name of person to whom information was communicated;

• Date and time of communication; and

• General review of information released.

Answering machines

Answering machines have become increasingly popular for use in small office settings. Although this method of access is appropriate, care must be taken to prevent delays in communicating critical clinical information. If the answering machine does not provide alternate access to the physician by direct use of a pager, the device must provide adequate information to the caller and allow the caller to leave a message. The following safeguards can minimize liability and patient frustration and protect physicians from allegations of abandonment.

First, advise patients in advance that an answering device is used when you are unavailable. Program the taped message to do the following:

• Provide an opening warning: if the situation is an emergency, direct the caller to the emergency department or paramedics;

• Provide ambulance information;

• Inform the patient when to expect a return call;

• Ask the caller to state his/her name and phone number, the date and time; and

• State the office hours and say when the office will re-open.

Be sure to use an answering device that accommodates a sufficient number of incoming calls and does not rewind or overwrite.

Automated telephone systems

Although convenient for the office practice, automated phone systems do not provide warm, empathetic, caring interaction. This can create confusion, anger and frustration for patients at the very onset of the communication.

While these systems are often discouraged in health care settings, if they are used, avoid long detailed messages that have multiple menu selections. And make sure the instructions are simple and clear.

Scheduling

Everyone needs to have the ability to schedule appointments. One thing I have noticed is that all the work we do to try and identify the exact reason for a visit often fails. The appointment types that were identified in *The Making of an Efficient Physician* relied on higher skill level schedulers. However, what we have concluded over the past four years is that a more simplified scheduling system is really more accurate than the more complex system we talked about in the first book. Sophisticated scheduling systems end up being very resource intensive and not very effective. Simplifying the scheduling process allows more flexibility in who can schedule; decreases the resource time in scheduling an appointment; and with a single appointment time, soothes the flow.

When the patient calls for an appointment, be sure to register any new patient. If you have open access, you will not need to worry about new patients not showing up for their visit. One of the benefits of an open access system is a decrease in the no-show rate. Registering patients over the phone will decrease the delay when they check in for their visit. After scheduling the appointment, it is important to remind patients to bring in their co-pay or any balance that is due, along with their insurance card. Helping patients prepare for the visit is very important. It is helpful to ask patients to fax in a copy of their insurance card, if possible, to enable your staff to verify their eligibility prior to the visit.

It is also the time to remind the patient to bring in all current medications. This will allow the support staff to accurately document the current medications as well as identify the refill date and prepare the refill paperwork for the physician to sign. This will reduce a future phone call and help reduce the physician's time trying to identify what medications a person is taking. Also remind patients to bring in their child's immunization record, if appropriate.

If the appointment is a follow-up from the emergency room or hospital, obtain the name of the hospital and make sure the discharge notes are ordered and on the chart before the visit.

Remind new patients of the location and thank them for calling.

Preparation

Taking a few minutes each day to prepare for the patients' visits will help your day run smoothly. Stock all rooms alike. Make sure each room is stocked at least once a day.

"AM huddles" take five minutes or so. The daily agenda is simple and includes three items:

- Is there any follow-up work from yesterday that needs to be completed?

- Are there any anticipated problems or challenges in today's schedule?

- Are there any problems with tomorrow's schedule that need to be corrected today?

This daily get-together is a great way to quickly share information with your team, thank people for the extra effort, answer questions and discuss concerns. It is obvious to a patient when the team is in sync, working together and when it is out of sync and chaotic.

Medical records

Unless you have an automated medical record or online chart notes, it is preferable to have medical records housed at each work unit. The delay in workflow caused by retrieving medical records as well as the increased support staff costs does not speak well for centralized medical records. Medical records should be part of many tasks, not an isolated task. If you are part of a large multispecialty practice where many different physicians are working out of the same medical record, consideration of an automated medical record or online chart notes should be a high priority.

Check in

The check-in function has become a "greeter" function in many office practices. If you have the technology in the exam rooms to take the patient directly to the exam room, it is preferable to patients. However, if you do not have this technology in the exam rooms, the greeter can verify demographic information, take a copy of the insurance card, if it was not faxed in prior to the visit, and verify the insurance via the medifax, roster or telephone. Work with your insurance companies to automate this procedure. More and more insurance companies are going online. Insurance information is directly input into the system either before the visit or while the patient is there so the face sheet can be printed off and given to the patient to verify and sign. At no time is the staff asking the patient personal question in front of other patients. Because of the even flow of patients coming in, there is no need for patients to sign in.

This is the time to collect all co-pays and old balances. If patients are reminded when they call for the visit, they will not be surprised when asked by the greeter for payment. Be sure to give the patient a receipt, stamp all checks and place any cash in the locked cash box.

The chart is prepared prior to the visit. Make sure each page of the chart has the patient's name and the date of service. The greeter attaches the new face sheet with the current phone number highlighted, the fee slip, labels to be used if necessary, and an insurance guide sheet to the front of the chart and the patient is ready to go to the exam room. Highlighting the phone number after verifying with the patient that it is correct will facilitate easy access for the physician or staff if they need to contact the patient in the future.

The insurance guide sheet is a form that identifies all pertinent information about each insurance plan. As the patient flows through the system, whomever touches the patient will have at their fingertips a list of phone numbers, carve-out procedures, referral expectations, formulary needs and any other information that will facilitate the care of each patient. The following form is a sample of an insurance guide sheet.

Insurance guide sheet

Customer Service # 1-800-XXX-XXXX

Members must be assigned to a PCP : PCPs generate all required referrals
This product is capitated: Encounter claim forms: No deductible

Eligibility / Benefits Verification:□	1-800-XXX-XXXX □	Auto Status
CoPays:□	Vary with Plan□	Check Card
Claims Processing:□□		Electronic
Referral / Prior Authorization □ Requirements:□ □ □□ □□	Complete form. For procedures listed on form prior □ authorizations is required.□	□Fax all prior authorizations to 1-XXX-XXX-XXXX. 24 hour turnaround. All others hand to patient to hand carry to appointment.
Ancillary Providers:□ □ □ □ □ □	• Laboratory Services□ • Radiology Services□ • CT MRI□ • Physical Therapy□ • Home Health □ • Durable Medical Equipment□ • Pharmacy□	• □XYZ Lab • □ABC Radiology • □ABC Radiology • □DEF PT • □Home Care XYZ • □DMC • □Pharmacy Group
Carve-Out Services:□ □	J- Codes, Immunizations, Newborn Care	
Provider Relations Contact:□	Jane Doe□	XXX-XXXX
Termination Requirements:□ □□ □ □□	• Member can disenroll at any time • Non-compliant patient Termination Fill out form	
Self-Referral Benefits□ □ □	Annual Well-Women Exam OB Care Mental Health Care	
Referrals□	Specialty Network	
Formulary□ □ □	Formulary Exceptions complete □ an Integrate Pharmacy Service □ Drug Request Form□	□Fax to 1-XXX-XXX-XXXX return response within 24 hours - no retro authorizations.
Service Standards□ □ □ □ □	• Preventive Care□ • Routine Visits□ • Symptomatic Visit□ • Urgent Visits□ • Emergent Visits□	30 days 7 days 3 days 24 hours patient to call 911
Education Opportunities□ 1-800-XXX-XXXX□ □	Body Mind□ Family Care□ Smoking Management□	Personal Safety Senior Health Disease management
Hospitals□	ABC Hospital	

Communication – front office to back

Because of the open architecture, it is easy for our staff in the back office to see when the patient is ready to move to the exam room. If you do not have the ability to see when a patient is ready, you will need to have a light system, beeper system or some other tool to let the back office know when the patient is ready.

Chapter 11

Process

Process function

The process function includes all tasks from rooming the patient until, but not including, check-out. Of the three positions, this needs the most medical skills. The other two positions are predominately clerical, however, having a medical assistant's background is helpful.

Preparing the patient

The more done during the rooming phase of the encounter, the shorter the visit is for the physician. Make sure the patient is ready when the physician enters the room. One good way to assure that staff consistently room patients appropriately is to develop a rooming criteria tool. The following page is an example of a rooming tool that works well in many clinics.

Rooming Criteria

Reason for visit	HT.	WT.	Head Circ.	BP.	Temp	Pulse	Resp	Vision	Gown	Expose area	Expose feet	Ck allergies	Ck phone #	Health maintenance forms	Immunization forms	Diabetic flow sheet	Chaperone
New CPE (includes P/P & Annuals)	X	X		X	X	X	X		after prov sees			X	X	X	X		X
Est. CPE (includes P/P & Annuals)	X	X		X	X	X	X		X			X	X	X	X		X
School/sports/PE	X	X		X	X	X	X	X	X			X	X	X	X		X
WCC	X	X		X	X	X	X		X			X	X	Age specific	X		
Chief Complaint					X					X		X	X	X	X		
Adult																	
Pain any system					X					X		X	X	X	X		
Respiratory		X		X	X	X	X					X	X	X	X		
Cardiac		X		X	X	X	X		X			X	X	X	X		
Dermatology				X	X					X		X	X	X	X		
Orthopedic				X	X					X		X	X	X	X		
Diabetic		X		X							X	X	X	X	X	X	
Children	X	X	<18m	3y+	X	X	X	5y+		X		X	X	X	X		
OMT				X									X	X	X		
Rechecks (depends on reason for recheck use above criteria)																	
Repeat Pap		X		X	X				X				X				X
Breast Check		X		X	X				X				X				X
Follow up < 3 wks				X									X				
Lab Only													X				

When taking a BP be sure to watch to see if the monometer reading returns to zero.

When weighing a patient be sure to zero the scale first.

Staff to document reason for visit – providers to obtain history.

As you develop your rooming tool, remember simplification. Too much detail or variation by type of visit will lead to more patients being roomed inappropriately. This tool can double as a training tool for new employees.

The first column of the tool lists the reason for the visit. We divided it into routine, acute or chief complaint and recheck visits. Across the top of the page are the categories of tasks. Each category acts as a reminder. An example is "expose feet," which is listed under diabetic visit. It has been found that if the staff will make sure the diabetic patient's feet are exposed, foot exams are completed and documented more often. The tool also reminds staff to make sure the chart has a diabetic flow sheet completed.

At the bottom of the Rooming Criteria tool you will note several reminders of basics that staff often forget.

Chaperoning

A few word about chaperoning during the physical exam. I have worked with physicians who do not believe it is ever necessary and others who will not see a patient without a chaperone. More and more it is becoming an issue because of the high number of lawsuits against physicians. Since many patients today choose their physician out of a directory, the relationship that used to develop between physician and patient has changed. To protect yourself, I would recommend at least giving your patients the option of whether or not they would like someone else in the room. Be sure to document their response in your notes.

If you choose to build the chaperoning task into your system, make sure it is value-added. Some clinics will have the medical assistant scribe as they do the exam. Others will have them filling out paperwork, preparing for tests or assisting the physician.

Remember it is not only needed when male physicians examine female patients. There have been many suits against female physicians, when examining female patients. The gender of the physician or the patient really doesn't matter. If you have a policy, treat everyone the same.

It is also important that you develop a system for notifying your medical assistant when you would like one of them to enter the room. Some clinics that use the medical assistant as a scribe do not need an alert since the assistant will always be present, however, most clinics need some type of alert system. If your support staff can easily see all the rooms, the easiest and least expensive alert is just to crack open the door. However, most rooms are not visible to the support staff, therefore, beepers, buzzers, light systems, or even telephones are tools that many clinics will use.

Communication tools

The following pages are copies of communication tools designed by physicians. The purpose of each is to document appropriately to meet all regulatory requirements. Efficiency also improves with good forms. While most routine exams are dictated, many acute visits are documented on the progress notes to decrease follow-up work and to cut costs of transcription.

Sample Pediatric Progress Note and Worksheet

┌   Patient Label   ┐

Name:_____
Date:_____
Age:_____

└ _____ ┘

Pediatric Progress Notes & Worksheet

CC (reason for visit)	Provider:
Current medications	Accompanied by:
	Allergies

S:

History _____

Social/Family: _____

ROS (review of system)

O:

Physical examination:
Ht:_____WT:_____HC:_____   T:_____ P:_____ R:_____ BP:_____
(%tile)_____(%tile)_____(%tile)_____

RN/LPN/MA:_____

N	AB			N	AB	
❑	❑	Gen. appearance_____		❑	❑	Heart_____
❑	❑	Head_____		❑	❑	Abdomen_____
❑	❑	Eyes_____		❑	❑	Nodes_____
❑	❑	Nose_____		❑	❑	G.U._____
❑	❑	L. Ear_____		❑	❑	Hips/Extremities_____
❑	❑	R. Ear_____		❑	❑	Spine_____
❑	❑	Oropharynx_____		❑	❑	Skin_____
❑	❑	Neck_____		❑	❑	Neuro_____
❑	❑	Lungs_____		❑	❑	Growth & Devel_____

Exam comments:_____

A:

Assessment_____

P:

Plan: Labs/X-Ray:_____

Meds:_____

Immunizations: ❑ DTaP ❑ DPT ❑ Polio ❑ MMR ❑ HIB ❑ Tetramune ❑ HepB ❑ Varicella
               ❑ Other:_____ ❑ Advised to bring in immunization records & dates
Return to office in _____ days/weeks/months/PRN
Signed:_____ ❑ Dictated ❑ Written Only
      (provider)
Comments/Counseling issues:_____

Visit time:_____ Counseling time:_____

Sample Adult Progress Note #1

Progress Notes

Time_____

Age_____ DOB_____ T_____ P_____ R_____ BP_____ Ht_____ Wt_____

CC_____LMP_____Pregnant?_____

Allergies_____ Last Tetanus_____

HPI_____ Medications_____

_____ _____

_____ _____

_____ _____

_____ _____

Past Medical History:_____

_____

Family History:_____

_____

Social History:_____

_____

ROS (pertinent note +/- findings):_____

_____

_____

Physical Exam

_____

_____

_____

_____

_____

_____

_____

Assessment:_____ Plan (Counseling Issues):_____

_____ _____

_____ _____

_____ _____

_____ _____

_____ _____

_____ _____

Visit Time_____Counseling Time_____   Signature_____ dictated_____

Progress Notes

Sample Adult Progress Note #2

Provider	Room	Date

Chief Complaint:

Age:_____   Wt:_____
BP:_____   HT:_____
P:_____   Temp:_____
R:_____   LMP:_____

HPI & ROS: (4+ elements)

Allergies:_____
Immunizations:_____
Tobacco:_____
EtOH:_____

Exam:

(Limited; affected area/organ and symptomatic related systems)

Meds:_____
_____
_____

General _____
HEENT _____
Neck _____
Heart _____
Lungs _____
Abdomen _____
Skin _____

Key: ✓ = Reviewed/Within Normal Limits)
Lab, X-Rays:

Diagnosis: _____

Plan:

-
-
-

Follow up: ❏ Prn   ❏ Other _____
❏ Call if worse or symptoms persist
❏ Call in 24-48 hours for lab results
❏ Other_____

Patient Name_____
Medical Record Number_____
PCP_____

Provider Signature
❏ Please file this note   ❏ Note dictated

Patient here with:
_____

From Virginia Mason Medical Center, Seattle. Used to decrease transcription costs for acute visits only. Used with permission.

The following waiver is used in many clinics to document the person's permission for leaving test results over the phone.

Contact with normal labs? Yes___ No___
Leave message on recorder? Yes___ No___
Leave message with another person? Yes___ No___
If yes with whom?_____
Phone number to call with results_____
Morning___ Afternoon____
Is it ok to call at work? Yes___ No ____ Work phone____ Ext. ____
Witness_____ Patient Signature_____
Date _____

Answering machines

There is much confusion as to what can or cannot be left on a patient's recorder. Not letting the staff leave messages causes tremendous rework. My staff's solution was to use the above waiver. It works well. We went back to basics and let the patient make the decision. Most patients are pleased to be asked and really appreciate being notified immediately of their test results. If the tests are abnormal, patients are asked to call the office.

This change dramatically reduced the number of outgoing calls, as well as, the delay in returning test results – since they only had to call once. In the past they would try for days to get hold of a patient, only to find out they had the wrong number or the patient was never home and they did not feel comfortable leaving a message. This way as soon as the test results are in, the patient is called, the tests are filed and the chart is put back in medical records. A small change that made a big difference!

Order worksheet

Another tool to help the physician communicate with both the patient and staff is the order worksheet. The following page is a sample of a tool we use in many of our clinics. As the physician is talking with the patient, he/she records on the worksheet the plan. This reminds the physician to address how test results are reported, if the waiver system is not in place. It also lists all the tests that were ordered as well as any referrals or nursing intervention needed. The back can be used for any instructions you may want to give to the patient. Remember patients only remember about 30 percent of what you tell them, so write it down. A few minutes of documentation will save hours of support staff time answering calls from patients who forgot what you said. We will discuss in the next chapter how the output function person will use this form.

Following the worksheet form you will find five other forms that are used to help physicians document appropriately and efficiently: the Summary of Care form meets the regulatory requirement of JCAHO; the Acute Care form, keeps the Summary of Care form from filling up with acute visits; the Immunization form; and two Health Maintenance forms. Remember forms are continually being updated and improved. As you read this book, these forms may already be outdated. Find similar ones that meet these needs.

Sample Order Worksheet

Order worksheet Date Ordered_____

TEST RESULTS		REFERRAL		
When:		Diagnosis:		
❑ Call patient w/ results	Phone:	Refer to:		
❑ Form letter	❑ Dictated letter	Symptoms/Findings:		
❑ Dictated letter to patient:	❑ Physician:			
❑ Results to be given	❑ Address:			
❑ To Pt. on f/u visit	❑ Other:			
❑ Automated call back	❑ Address	Send records ❑ yes ❑ no		
❑ No action required	❑ Date reported:	TO:		
VISIT FOLLOW-UP				
❑ Return visit in:	Provider:			
❑ Visit type brief, extended, etc.				
❑ List as personal physician				
❑ Computer reminder (tickler) for when:				

When sequencing is important, use a number in the box rather than a check

LABORATORY						CARDIOLOGY LABS		ICD
Routine	Stat	Routine	Stat	Routine	Stat	❑ ECG Age Ht Wt		
❑ CBC w/ differ.		❑ Chem. profile		❑ Serum sodium		❑ Send w/ Pt ❑ Send Previous Study		
❑ Estrogen level		❑ Cocci Serology		❑ Strep culture		❑ Cardiac Meds:		
❑ Chem 24 (SMAC)		❑ Digoxin		❑ Theophyline		❑ Treadmill: ❑ MD ❑ RN		
❑ Chem 7		❑ Dilantin		❑ VDRL		❑ Type ❑ Reason		
❑ TSH		❑ FSH		❑ Pregnancy test		❑ ECHO ❑ Routine ❑ Stress ❑ LV Mass		
❑ TSH/T3		❑ Glucose finger		❑ Sputum Gram		❑ Reason		
❑ T4 Free +T7		❑ Glycohemoglobin		❑ RBC/Virol		❑ Holter ❑ 24 Hr. ❑ 48 hr. ❑ Reason:		
❑ UA/C&S		❑ HDL Cholesterol		❑ Microalbumin Dip		❑ Event Rec. Symptoms:		
❑ Urine Dipstick		❑ Lithium		❑ Lipid Profile		❑ 24 hour BP Monitoring ❑ Other		
❑ Urine Micro Albumin		❑ Pap Smear		❑		**PULMONARY LAB**		
❑ PT/INR		❑ Protime/INR.		❑		❑ FVC (Only): With DB (no inhaler last 4 hours)		
❑ PTT		❑ PSA		❑		❑ PFTS - Pre/Post BD		
❑ Mono spot		❑ RA Factor		❑		❑ 02 Sat ❑ Peak Flow ❑ Other		
❑ Hepatitis Profile		❑ Sed Rate		❑		**MICROBIOLOGY**		
❑ Hemoccult		❑ Serum Calcium		ICD		Culture ❑ Wound (location		
❑ ANA/Profile		❑ Serum Magnesium				Vaginal: ❑ Wet ❑ KOH ❑ UA Dipstick		
❑ B12/Folate		❑ Serum Potassium				Stool: ❑ O&P ❑ Set ❑ Path ❑ CDT ❑ w/ Diff		
RADIOLOGY		REASON	FAX	ICD		Sputum: ❑ Routine ❑ Induced		
❑ Chest PA & LAT						❑ Call Result ❑ C&S if Purulent		
❑ Abdominal screen:	Series							
❑ Sinus Screen:	Series					**CULTURES**		Source
❑ UGI SBFT		❑ Prep				❑ GC Screen ❑ Throat/Strep ❑ Urine		
❑ BE:		❑ Prep				❑ Chlamydia EIA ❑ Ova & Parasites ❑ Wound		
❑ Sine:						❑ HSV ❑ Stool		
❑ Mammogram		❑ Prep				❑ Culture: ❑ Bact ❑ AFB ❑ Fung		
❑ US		❑ Prep				❑ Culture: ❑ Bact ❑ AFB ❑ Fung		
❑ Nuclear Medicine:						**IMMUNIZATIONS**		
❑ Venous Duplex:						❑ TD ❑ DtP ❑ OPV/IPV ❑ HIB ❑ Acellular Pertussis		
❑ MRI: ❑ w/Gadolinium ❑ Prep						❑ Tetramune ❑ Varicella ❑ PPD ❑ Cocci Skin Tes		
❑ CT: ❑ w/Contrast ❑ Prep						❑ Pneumo ❑ Influenza		
❑ w/o Contrast						**NURSING**		
❑ Other						❑ Cerumen Removal: RLB ❑ Foot Care		
OTHER STUDIES						❑ Chem Stick BG ❑ Audio Screen		
❑ Fecal Coag		❑ Flex Sig:				❑ Oximetry ❑ Rest ❑ Exercise ❑ Vision Screen		
❑ Hearing Aid Eval	❑ Audiogram	❑ Tymp				❑ Peak Flow ❑ MDI Inhaler		
❑ Vaginal Pap	❑ Previous Atypical					❑ Anticoagulation Tx ❑ Wound Care:		
❑ EMBX	❑ Reason					❑ Social Work: ❑ Education		
						❑ Home Health ❑ Other Education		
						❑ DM ❑ BP ❑ HIV ❑ Other:		
						❑ Handout(s) ❑ Other		

Sample of Summary of Care Form

Summary of Care

Daytime Phone:_____Pharmacy Phone:_____
Allergies:_____

#	Chronic Illnesses	Onset	Continuing Medications	Start	Stop

Prior Surgeries/Hospitalizations	Date	Social History/Habits	Date
		Occupation:	
		Tobacco:	
		ETOH:	
		Illicit Drugs:	
		Living Will:	
		Health Maint/Immuniz. UTD:	
		Check Up Visit:	
		Other:	
		Next of Kin:	

Significant Family History:
Father
Mother
Siblings:
Grandparents
Other:

Sample Acute Care Form

Acute Care

Date	Acute Problems	Treatment	Recurrence			

Sample Immunization Form

Immunization Administration Record

Name	
Birthdate	**I.D. Number**

Allergies:_____

Previous Adverse Immunization Reaction:_____

"I have read or have had explained to me the information contained in the Vaccine Information Pamphlet about the following disease(s) and vaccine(s): polio (live and killed), Diphtheria, Tetanus, Pertussis, Measles, Mumps, Rubella singly or in combination, Haemophilus Influenzae type b, Hepatitis B, Pneumovax, Influenza and Varicella. I have had a chance to ask questions that were answered to my satisfaction. I believe I understand the benefits and risks of the vaccine(s) and request the the vaccine(s) indicated on this form be given to me or the person named on this health record for whom I am authorized to make this request."

Vaccine	Date Admin	Patient Age	Signature of person to receive Vaccine or person authorized to make request	Vaccine manufacturer	Vaccine Lot number	Site given	Signature of Vaccine administrator
DTP/DT 1						LVL RVL / LD RD	
DTP/DT 2						LVL RVL / LD RD	
DTP/DT 3						LVL RVL / LD RD	
DTP/DTaP 4						LD RD	
DTP/DTaP 5						LD RD	
Td						LD RD	
Td						LD RD	
OPV/IPV 1						ORAL / SQ: LD RD	
OPV/IPV 2						ORAL / SQ: LD RD	
OPV/IPV 3						ORAL / SQ: LD RD	
OPV/IPV 4						ORAL / SQ: LD RD	
MMR 1						LSQ RSQ	
MMR 2						LSQ RSQ	
Measles						LSQ RSQ	
Hib 1						LVL RVL / LD RD	
Hib 2						LVL RVL / LD RD	
Hib 3						LVL RVL / LD RD	
Hib 4						LD RD	
Hep B 1						LVL RVL / LD RD	
Hep B 2						LVL RVL / LD RD	
Hep B 3						LVL RVL / LD RD	
PneumovaX						LVL RVL / LD RD	
Varicella 1						LSQ RSQ	
Varicella 2						LSQ RSQ	
Influenza						LVL RVL / LD RD	

❑ Immunization/Medical Record Requested

Date_____

Skin Tests

Test	Date Given	Signature of Provider	Date Read	Result	Test	Date Given	Signature of Provider	Date Read	Result

Male Health Maintenance Form

Adult Male Patient

Routine Health Screening & Immunizations

Name_____

Medical record #_____DOB_____

Advance Directives: ❏ Yes (place copy on chart) ❏ No

Screening Recommendations*

Screening Test/Procedure	Patient Risk	Screening Age	Screening Frequency	Last Screening (obtain from patient)	Year: Age:	Year: Age:	Year: Age:	Year: Age:	Year: Age:
Rectal Exam (Colon Cancer Screen)	Avg	≥50	Annual						
	High	See MIH CPG							
Stool for Occult Blood (Colon Cancer Screen)	Avg	≥50	Annual						
	High	See MIH CPG							
Flex. Sigmoidoscopy (Colon Cancer Screen)	Avg	≥50	q 3-5 yrs						
	High	See MIH CPG							
PSA* (Prostate Cancer Screen)	Avg	≥50	Annual						
	High	≥40	Annual						

*Provide patient with "Patient Information on Prostate Cancer Screening" for informed decision on risk/benefits of prostate screening.

LDL & HDL Lipid Profile (CAD Screen)	Avg LDL<130 HDL>40	Early 20's	One Time for baseline level						
		35-75	Every 5 years						
	high	35-75	Annual						
Immunizations									
Pneumococcal	Avg	>65	One time dose consider re-vaccination every 6-10 years						
	high	all ages	max q 7 yrs						
Influenza	Avg	≥65	Annual						
	high	all ages	Annual						
Td Booster	all	all ages	q 10 yrs						
Tuberculosis Screen for risk factors	Avg	all ages	Screen q 1-5 years for high risk						
	high	all ages	Annual						
Anticipatory Guidance	Provide age appropriate counseling: smoking, alcohol, diet, exercise, sexual health, safety, etc.			During any office visit					

* Routine Health Screening Recommendations are guidelines to assist in the provision of preventive health services. They are not meant to be exhaustive nor comprehensively inclusive and should in no way be used to overrule clinician's judgement as it related to individual cases.

O = ordered   PR = Patient Refused   P = Pend to later date   DE = Done Elsewhere

Developed by Mercy Family Health Clinic, Phoenix. Used with permission.

Female Health Maintenance Form

Adult <u>Female</u> Patient

Routine Health Screening & Immunizations

Name_____

Medical record #_____DOB_____

Advance Directives: ❑ Yes (place copy on chart)   ❑ No

Screening Recommendations*									
Screening Test/Procedure	Patient Risk	Screening Age	Screening Frequency	Last Screening (obtain from patient)	Year: Age:	Year: Age:	Year: Age:	Year: Age:	Year: Age:
Rectal Exam (Colon Cancer Screen)	Avg	≥50	Annual						
	High	See MH CPG							
Stool for Occult Blood (Colon Cancer Screen)	Avg	≥50	Annual						
	High	See MH CPG							
Flex. Sigmoidoscopy (Colon Cancer Screen)	Avg	≥50	q 3-5 yrs						
	High	See MH CPG							
Clinical Breast Exam (Breast Cancer Screen)	Avg	18-39 >40	q 1-3 yrs annual						
	High	18-34 >35	q 1-3 yrs annual						
Mammogram (Breast Cancer Screen)	Avg	40-49 ≥50	q other year annual						
	High	>35	annual						
LDL & HDL Lipid Profile (CAD Screen)	Avg LDL<130 HDL>40	Early 20's	One Time for baseline level						
		45-75	Every 5 years						
	High	45-75	Annual						
Pap Smear (Cervical Cancer Screen)	Avg	Onset sexual activity or by age 18	q 1-3 yrs (annual until after 3 normal consecutive pap smears						
		Post-hysterectomy for benign process	No routine screening (if 3 most recent and consecutive pap smears normal							
	High	Any age	q 3-8 months						
Bimanual Pelvic Exam	Avg	Onset sexual activity or by age 18	q 1-3 yrs						
		Post-hysterectomy for benign process	q 3-5 yrs						
	High	Any age	q 6-12 months						
Immunizations									
Pneumococcal	Avg	>65	One time dose consider re-vaccination every 6-10 years						
	High	All ages	max q 7 yrs						
Influenza	Avg	≥65	Annual						
	High	All ages	Annual						
Td Booster	All	All ages	q 10 yrs						
Tuberculosis Screen for risk factors	Avg	All ages	Every 1-5						
	High	All ages	Annual						
Anticipatory Guidance	Provide age appropriate counseling: smoking, alcohol, diet, exercise, sexual health, safety, etc.			During any and all office visits					

* Routine Health Screening Recommendations are guidelines to assist in the provision of preventive health services. They are not meant to be exhaustive nor comprehensively inclusive and should in no way be used to overrule clinician's judgment as it relatedsto individual cases.

O = ordered   PR = Patient Refused   P = Pend to later date   DE = Done Elsewhere

Developed by Mercy Family Health Clinic, Phoenix. Used with permission.

Coding is a team responsibility

Only the physician knows what was done in the exam room. It is the responsibility of the physician to determine the appropriate CPT and ICD-9 codes. Learning how to code appropriately seems like a monumental task, however, the physicians who have taken the time to learn the basics, have much better reimbursement than those who allow a staff member to choose the code. The only exception would be a certified coder who is coding from your documentation. However, in ambulatory care, this is a major delay in the process and does not allow for payment at time of service. It also adds unnecessary cost to your practice. I like to remind physicians that they made it through medical school and they can learn to code. You can be the best physician in the world and if you do not code and document what you do appropriately, you may not get paid for your services.

Also be sure to ask your patients to complete a waiver statement if you are ordering tests not covered by their insurance. Without the waiver, you are not able to bill the patient.

Superbills

It is important that physicians have updated superbills to code from. It is also important that someone in your office stays current on all billing changes. It is helpful if you attend a coding class annually that is put on by the professional organization of your specialty. Your superbill should be a tool to help you code. Each physician in our clinics is given an *Easy-Coder* book along with an information sheet to help them code to the fifth digit. On codes like diabetes, the specificity of your coding is important. Therefore, because there are too many codes to put on the superbill, our information sheet will list the page in the *Easy-Coder* book to look at to choose the appropriate code.

Hospital charges

It is important that hospital charges are keyed in on a daily basis. The following hospital charge slip has worked well to help physicians stay current on hospital charges. This form is given to the desk assistant as soon as the physician returns from the hospital or the next working day, if it was in the evening or weekend. The physician annotates the charge on the appropriate day and the assistant keys in the charge and hands the form back to the physician. This form has helped our physicians improve their hospital billing compliance.

Sample Hospital Charge Slip

Hospital Charge Slip

Patient's Name_____ ❏ New   ❏ Established

Hospital: ❏ ❏ ❏

Diagnosis:_____ Physician:

A (Admit)	1. Ltd	(99221)	**C** (Consult)	1. Ltd.	(99251)	**ER** (Emerg.)	1. Ltd	(99281)
	2. Mod.	(99222)		2. Mod.	(99252)		2. Mod.	(99282)
	3. Comp.	(99223)		3. Comp.	(99253)		3. Comp.	(99283)
				4. H. Comp	(99254)		4. H. Comp.	(99284)

HV (Hosp. Visit)			**NHA** (Nursing Home Admit)			**NH** (Nursing Home Visit)		**SA** (Surgical Assist)
1. Ltd.	(99231)		1. Ltd.	(99301)		1. Ltd.	(99311)	**D** (Discharge)
2. Mod.	(99232)		2. Mod.	(99302)		2. Mod.	(99312)	**HC** (House Call)
3. Comp.	(99233)		3. Comp.	(99303)		3. Comp.	(99313)	1. Ltd. (99351)
								2. Mod. (99352)
								3. Comp. (99353)

Month:_____199

1	2	3	4	5	6	7
8	9	10	11	12	13	14
15	16	17	18	19	20	21
22	23	24	25	26	27	28
29	30	31				

Documentation

Before moving on to the next patient, be sure and complete your documentation. The chart can then be filed. It is far easier to pull a chart from medical records than to look for a chart stacked in someone's office.

Automation makes sense here!

The entire office visit could be streamlined with automation. The manual system most of us are using is very inefficient and resource intensive. Having an electronic medical record networked to the ancillary facilities, pharmacies, hospitals, insurance companies as well as other physicians in your area, could allow you to work more efficiently with less support and better service to your patients. Such automation is close. Many organizations around the country have been working on these systems for years. Without automation and with the increased need to see more with less, many physicians may not survive.

Transcription

Transcription is costly, but the tradeoffs are even more costly. Notes are illegible, hand writing long notes is very time-consuming and documentation becomes a constraint. There is hope for the voice-activated systems. However, until you have these tools, the best tool we have today is to develop templates that will decrease both the transcription time and your dictation time. If you send out your transcription, it really does not save any transcription cost since you are usually charged by number of lines. If you have in-house transcription, developing templates to dictate from will dramatically decrease your transcriptionist's time and costs.

Communicate in writing

Do not interrupt each other during the day. Use the "AM Huddle " to review your day, then as things arise, jot down notes to each other. Also do not let your staff interrupt you while you are with a patient unless it is truly an emergency. An interruption in the middle of the visit will not only slow down the visit and throw you off schedule, it will make the patient feel very unimportant. If a physician is calling, let him/her decide if you need to be interrupted. Often times a callback is sufficient.

e-mail

This technology is a wonderful way to communicate. However, you must remember that whatever goes over e-mail is no longer confidential. Many organizations use e-mail technology internally to manage messages.

Transition to the output function

Having a second support staff person working in the back with the physician allows the physician to directly transition the patient to the desk assistant. Since the physician has written down all the orders, there is no need to orally repeat the plan. The desk assistant can use the order sheet to begin the discharge task of the encounter.

Chapter 12

Output

Output function

The third function, output, encompasses tasks from discharge through follow-up. By using medical assistants in all three positions, you will have maximum flexibility. While each position has distinct tasks, the key to the success of this model is cross-training. When something needs to be done, whoever is available can do it – including the physician.

Discharge

When the exam portion of the visit is complete, either the physician or staff will walk the patient out to the desk assistant who is usually across from the exam room. At this point the paperwork is handed to the desk assistant and the remainder of the visit is completed.

Usually the first task is the discharge task. The medical assistant will review all the orders from the worksheet to make sure the patient understands everything and has no further questions. Reviewing the orders with the patient is important in assuring that nothing was missed that could cause a call back to the office or additional rework. After the orders are completed, a copy of the order sheet is given to the patient.

The three main tasks are done at this point: scheduling a follow-up appointment if applicable; completing the referral paperwork and calling or faxing the authorization information; and keying in the charges.

Follow-up appointment

Remember to use the dr. request appointment type and not to book the appointment on high demand days – unless of course that is the patient's preference.

Referrals

We have found that working with the insurance companies enables us to improve our referral process. As we studied the process, it was interesting to note the number of referrals that could have been done when the patient was in the clinic. However, at that time, our system did not allow for this since a separate person in a separate area did the referrals. By moving the task back to the desk assistant, we not only saved costs, we also decreased delays in referrals by weeks. Another benefit was that since the desk medical assistant had built a relationship with the patient, she was much more responsive to the follow-up on authorizations that had to be called in. Patients are much happier with the process. Staff are much happier because their volume of calls has dramatically decreased. It was a win-win for everyone.

Charge entry

As mentioned before, coding is a team effort. While the physician's responsibility for coding is the ICD-9 and CPT, as well as identifying the correct code for each ancillary charge, the desk nurse is responsible for checking for modifiers and reviewing the charge ticket for any errors. Since we also made the medical assistants responsible for correcting all errors, the error rate has gone from 65 percent to less than 5 percent. This is one indicator that we measure weekly and share the results with all the teams.

With the physician close to the charge entry point, if questions arise they can be answered on the spot. Keying charges at the time of the service has many advantages.

Errors decrease, accounts receivable improves and patients are happier knowing what the charge actually is and not being surprised when they receive a bill.

Test verification

If test results make it to the physician's desk, they usually get to the patient. However, problems occur when the test results never come back. Unless you have a system in place to track all tests and assure the results were returned to the office, you are setting yourself up for legal problems.

In our system we use the order sheet as a tickler file. However, this is definitely an area for automation.

Results reporting

By using the waiver system we talked about before, this becomes a very easy task. However, there are still many patients who request written response with the actual lab values. For these patients a tri-fold form letter is helpful. By using the tri-fold form, you eliminate the cost of an envelope and yet you can staple the form shut to assure confidentiality.

Many clinics, however, have gone to an automated response system. Patients find it easy to use and really appreciate being able to dial in at their convenience to retrieve their test results.

How physicians affect flow

As we mentioned before, physicians drive workflow in the office practice. There are very few tasks that do not affect the physician in one way or another. Therefore, when the physician is out of the office, most workflow comes to a halt. If you do not believe this to be true, look at a physician's office the day before he/she comes back from vacation and you will notice a stack of work waiting for him/her to return. The same thing happens during the day in many practices. At the end of the day physicians have a pile of work on their desks, They will stay late, review it, handle what needs to be handled and then pass it back to the assistant to be completed the following day. Now the medical assistant has to take time out of today's schedule to do work that could have been given to her yesterday had the physician been using the continuous flow principle.

Handle messages as they come in. Dictate as you go. Never batch work to do later. Using these simple techniques, your days will be shorter, work life will be better and your productivity will improve.

Chapter 13

Financial picture

Breakeven strategy

Many hospital-affiliated primary care practices are losing up to $120,000 per physician per year. It is a difficult challenge with the reimbursement decreasing to breakeven to meet the compensation expectations of the physicians. By using MGMA benchmarking, you can determine where the problem lies in your practice. Operating expenses should be compared in five categories:

- Salaries and benefits;

- Supplies and services;

- Building and occupancy;

- Professional fees and services; and

- Other expenses.

Comparing these categories with the MGMA benchmarks will identify areas of concern. The following discussion identifies tools for dealing with these concerns.

Increase net medical revenue

Decreased physician productivity reflects low gross revenue numbers. If gross revenue numbers are in range, high contractual adjustments may result in low net revenue. While net revenue per physician is the benchmark of concern, visits, RVUs and hours in clinic are all tools to help us identify the cause of low net revenue.

Control costs

Cost accounting is the process for determining the cost of products and services associated with the delivery of patient care. The end result is to provide meaningful cost information to allow better utilization of resources, as well as the ability to benchmark against other similar practices. This will support operational improvements and demonstration of value by measuring and tracking the actual cost of patient care delivery. Most physicians do not have sophisticated cost accounting systems, however, understanding the major expense categories will allow you to benchmark against MGMA data. The most common categories are:

•   Non-provider salary and benefits;

•   Supply costs;

•   Building and occupancy costs; and

•   Other.

Benchmarking

•   Some helpful indicators to measure over time are:

•   Revenue per physician;

•   Filled hours;

•   Total visits;

- Revenue per visit;

- Non-provider cost as a percent of net revenue;

- Cost per visit;

- Provider compensation as a percent of net revenue; and

- Gain (loss) per provider.

Collections and income

Inform new patients of your billing/collection policies. It is helpful to include them in your New Patient Packet. This communication phase is where you can make or break your collection program. Most problems between individuals are a result of lack of communication. You must make sure your office is communicating your policies and the patient understands them.

Obtain accurate information up front. Keying in the information while interviewing the patient is the most accurate way to do this. Print the form, have the patient review the information and sign the document.

As noted previously, collect co-pays and any old balances up front. Remind patients when they schedule their appointment about their co-pay and or balance due.

Daily cash receipts and keying of superbills should be done by two separate individuals to assure cash controls.

Charges and cash collections should be posted to patients' accounts at time of service. However, physicians must complete the superbill in order for staff to complete the process. Timely posting of cash and charges will increase accuracy and efficiency of the reconciliation process and financial reporting. It will also give your staff the opportunity to ask for payment if appropriate.

Annually update your charge master or superbill. This will ensure you are current.

Checks should be restrictively endorsed upon receipt, not during the reconciliation process.

A few words about cash controls

We never want to think that one of our employees may be dishonest. However, embezzlement is a major problem in private practices. By proactively establishing good cash handling and charge controls systems, you will not have to worry.

If you have one person who determines charges, collects cash, prepares the daily deposit, records the daily revenue and enters charges into the billing system, your system is at risk for potential misuse of cash. The major problem is the lack of segregation of duties; i.e., allowing the same person to perform all cash- and charge-related activities. Internal control is compromised when one employee is given authority to determine charges and accept cash, as well as monitor the subsequent accounting entries. It is relatively easy for an employee to understate collections and not charge a friend for medical services, that were rendered. Physicians should make the charge selections on the superbill identifying the appropriate CPT code as well as the appropriate ICD-9 codes.

Daily bank deposits are a must. Allowing cash to accumulate invites individuals to "borrow" from the available funds for personal use; i.e., planning to return the funds before the cash is deposited.

A proper monthly bank reconciliation is imperative. This is where discrepancies should be identified. A supervisor needs to reconcile the superbills against the schedule to verify that the charges accurately reflect the services rendered. Superbills should be numbered and reconciled on a daily basis. A dishonest employee could possibly steal the last package of superbills in a shipment, use them as patient receipts, subsequently preparing a second bill for a smaller amount and pocketing the difference. Further, the possibility exists that employees could provide stolen payment receipt documents to patients for subsequent use as verification of payment. Two individuals should check bank deposits. And always maintain an audit trail.

Quality indicators

We keep hearing that "you can't manage what you don't measure." Indicators are one form of measurement that can be linked to quality efforts. An indicator is a quantitative measure of a process or outcome. Indicators must be explicitly defined and lend themselves to accurate measurement over time.

Choose indicators in areas such as service, appropriateness and finance. Only pick a few because of the time it takes to gather and compile the data. Examples could be:

*   Service – Percent of patients rating the overall service as "Excellent";

*   Appropriateness – Immunization rate of 2-year olds; and

*   Financial – Outpatient cost per visit.

If your results do not meet your expectations, how do you develop a process improvement program? The next chapter provides some suggestions.

Chapter 14

Quality improvement

Continuous quality improvement

Continuous quality improvement (CQI) is a set of tools and techniques used to increase the value of work. The most important elements are:

- Data driven;

- Team approach;

- Process analysis;

- Customer focused;

- Increased empowerment of front-line workers; and

- Reduction of non-real work or waste in the system.

A simple model for improvement asks three questions:

- What are you trying to accomplish?

- How will you know if a change is an improvement?

- What change could you try that you believe will result in improvement?

You must have the ability to test your ideas. Don't make major changes without testing elements of the change first. Do short tests – one hour, one day or maybe one week. Learn first, then implement the change.

Example: Objective: Reduce wait time in reception area; increase patient availability in exam room.

Idea: If the assistants who room patients are at the reception area, they can greet patients and take them directly to the exam room. Test your idea.

Process: Patients are roomed in next available room. Roomers are stationed in reception area and patients are roomed immediately when an exam room is available.
Data collection: Measure the length of time in the reception area. Also measure patient satisfaction with the new process. Try it for a day and then ask, what did we learn? Revise the process based on the test results.

Take personal responsibility for quality

• Make a commitment to never-ending improvement.

• Honor your commitments.

• Make a daily "to do" list.

• Lead when a leader is needed.

• Define excellence for yourself.

• Be part of the solution.

• Admit your mistakes.

• Do your part in the group effort.

• Learn to say "I'm sorry."

• Strive for zero defects.

• Take charge of morale.

- Inspire trust.

- Offer suggestions.

- Look for opportunities in losses or mistakes.

- Accept revisions as proof that someone cares.

- Don't gossip or spread rumors.

The purpose of collecting data is to generate information

Data are facts – information is the answer to a question. Plan for data collection by answering a few questions:

- What question do we need to answer? Asking the right question implies knowledge of the process.

- What tools do we need to collect the data?

- Where in the process can we get the data?

- How can we collect the data with minimum effort and minimum chance of error?

- When possible, use data that already exists. Simplify data collection efforts. Collect data before and after a quality improvement effort.

- Plot data over time. It normally takes multiple small changes to meet your aim. However, improvements can be noted with as little as one change. As you make changes, measure the performance and plot the data over time. You can learn much more about your performance by observing trends and patterns in simple time series charts.

- Focus on measures of service directly related to your aim.

- Use sampling. It is not necessary to have data on every patient or every service experience in your system. Appropriate sampling procedures should be developed to minimize the cost of data collection and measurement. For example, measure every fifth patient or all patients for one day.

- Integrate measures into routine processes. Whenever possible, collect useful data as part of the normal performance of a process. Develop simple data recording forms that are integrated into the job.

Chapter 15

Tying it all together

You can make a difference

If decreased reimbursement, increased costs, increased regulatory controls and increased workload are forcing you to question whether or not you should continue to practice medicine, try some of the suggestions from the book. It will make a positive difference. If we all work together, continually looking for new and more efficient ways to care for our patients, we can improve health care and return to the days when it was gratifying to take care of patients.

Now is the time to take control

It is essential that physicians become active participants in the improvement of processes in their office practice. Improved efficiency results in improved productivity, greater capacity to provide services, less frustration and much greater satisfaction.

Patients are demanding that we improve our service and become more accessible. Many physicians believe they are already working beyond capacity. The only answer is to adopt the real-time work philosophy, open up capacity and begin to look at your work in a new way.

This book provides guidance for improving office efficiency. It will assist you in gaining extra productivity and daily capacity to provide care without increasing resources. This is accomplished by reallocating existing resources away from non-value-added activities toward those that really matter to both patients and physicians alike. By examining how patients move through the office, wasteful steps or procedures can be identified and eliminated.

Establishing aims and measures

The first step toward improvement is to set clear aims. What do you want to accomplish? What do you want your practice to look like? What do your patients want your practice to look like? The creation of aims requires the availability of useful measures to monitor your office system and your progress.

How will you know if a change is an improvement?

When you make a change in your office, you need to measure to see if the change actually improved the process. You also need to ask your patients if the change added value to their visit. Measures should not be burdensome for your staff. Keep it simple. Ask only a few patients. They will let you know right away if the change made a positive impact on their visit.

Observation is the greatest tool

Spend one day observing what goes on in your office. Sit with the schedulers, watch your staff do a referral, get involved. Not only will you identify constraints, you will have a better idea of how your actions affect all processes in the office. If you have a partner, use the day to follow a patient through the system. It is eye opening to see what we put our patients through. Key into staff's body language, tone of voice – they are your marketing team. Make sure the image they portray to the public is what you want.

Key changes for improving office efficiency

Adopting the following five key changes in your practice will show dramatic improvements in efficiency very quickly without much work. Keep in mind the guiding principles found in this book.

Preparation

Taking the time to prepare for the day is invaluable. Try an "AM huddle" where you and your staff meet for five minutes every morning to review the schedules for yesterday, today and tomorrow. This gives you the opportunity to follow up on any loose ends from yesterday and plan for tomorrow. When reviewing today's schedule, inform each other of anything out of the ordinary that may need to be done prior to each visit. Make sure that tomorrow's schedule is not full of errors. Note patients who are in the hospital or were seen yesterday and were not taken off the schedule.

When patients call in, begin preparing for the visit. Inform them of what they need to bring with them. Example would be insurance card, all medications (this dramatically decreases medication misspelling, as well as wrong doses. It also allows you to see when they are due to be renewed and you can give the patient a new script so they will not be calling in next week for a refill.

Don't forget to have the patient, room and paperwork ready when the patient arrives.

Standardization – decrease unnecessary variation

Standardizing processes is central to reducing unintended variation in your practice. Minimizing variation among staff, particularly providers, allows other staff to anticipate next steps in the process, thereby reducing time and need for communication between steps.

Having clear written policies and procedures allows staff to work for any provider. When rooms are stocked alike and needed equipment is in each room, the exam room never becomes the barrier.

Standardizing and minimizing your supply list will add to decreased supply cost if you maintain a par level inventory system. Par level inventory systems simply tell you when to order – keeping you from becoming a warehouse for old supplies.

Reduce rework

The easiest way to reduce rework is to do today's work today or "real-time" work.

Having an open access system where patients are seen on the day they call simplifies the scheduler's job, decreases the no-show rates and enhances positive patient satisfaction. By scheduling all patients the same length of time (usually your average visit time), this allows for a continuous flow of work for the staff. This allows them the time needed to complete each task, resulting in less rework.

Synchronizing tasks involving patient, provider, equipment and information is key to improving office efficiency. Timing of all steps in a process, such as patient flow, should be referred back to a clearly defined point in time. A critical example of office synchronization is getting appointments started on time. Late starts consume valuable resources, cause further downstream delays, and discourage staff.

Negotiate next steps – follow-up

While the patient is in the office, address the follow-up plan. Example: Explain when and how test results will be communicated back to the patient. This will not only decrease incoming calls, but will also decrease rework.

Put the treatment plan in writing. Many appointments are needed because of non-compliance. Remember, patients only remember 30 percent of what is told to them at the time of the visit. This will also decrease unnecessary phone calls to the office.

Recommend a good home care book like *Take Care of Yourself* by Donald M. Vickery, MD, and James F. Fries, MD. This will help decrease unnecessary visits and calls.

Manage your day

Days seldom turn out as planned – schedules change, staff call in sick, providers get called to the hospital. You must plan for the unexpected. Contingency plans need to be used when there is a temporary mismatch of supply and demand.

Efficient offices also understand constraints and recognize that in health care, the constraint is often the physician. These offices ensure that rooms and equipment are always available, and attempt to direct all unnecessary work away from the constraint. Everyone in the process works to the highest level of his/her license. However, as the day unfolds, people must be flexible enough to do what is needed to get the work completed efficiently and effectively. Teamwork and cross-training are the keys to working past constraints with minimal staffing levels and without compromising care.

Conclusions

When you follow the principles identified in this book, your office practice will run much smoother. You will have happy patients and a stable staff to help you improve the long-term viability of your practice. Creating an efficient office allows you to leave at the end of the day satisfied and assured that there will be a tomorrow.